The Modern Guide to Sex

GEORGIA GRACE

Harper *by* Design

*Dedicated to
everyone who learnt
about pleasure from
the shower head*

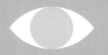

How do you feel?

I ask this of every person who sits across from me for our first session together. The answer is always the same. *Nervous*.

Clients come to me for help with their sex concerns. Often, they've never spoken about it with anyone before, let alone with a complete stranger. They're worried they are 'unfixable' or broken or abnormal. They might've tried a few things over the years but have finally decided to see a professional about it, and now they're nervous – and I can see it in their bodies too. Their posture is tight and small, their breath shallow, gaze averted, voice wavering.

And maybe you feel that way too? So before we go any further – how do *you* feel to be here, to be with me and this book? How do you feel physically, mentally, emotionally and sexually? Perhaps you are reading this book because you've never been taught about pleasure and you want some tools, or maybe you can't shut off distracting thoughts during sex. Maybe you want to have your first ever orgasm, or you're in a long-term relationship and your partner has voiced a concern and you're now worried you're incompatible. Maybe

sex is already great and you want to make it even better, or maybe you're a self-proclaimed sex freak and your bookshelf is a slut for sex ed.

Regardless of what brought you to this book, I'm glad you're here. You are not alone in the questions you have about sex. In fact, rarely does a sex question surprise me. I've seen, heard and experienced a lot. And I've noticed that we are all more alike than we may think (or want to believe). There are differences in what turns us on, what sparks anxiety, what intrigues or disgusts us. But a few things I know for sure: at some point we've all had a sex question, we've all wondered if a desire was normal and we've all been confused by our bodies.

As I was growing up, I didn't always 'get' sex. My attraction to all people regardless of their gender was disorienting, but I've always been curious about sex. Sex ed was limited and my friends knew as little as I did. The internet offered ten tips to 'blow his mind' and not much else, books only just scratched the surface and largely focused on cis heterosexual experiences, and trial and error only got me so far.

4

Like so many of us, I didn't receive the accurate, sex-positive, pleasure-focused and inclusive information I so desperately wanted.

Then I discovered the field of somatic sexology. It's a therapeutic practice that explores human sexuality through an awareness of the mind and the body – and I wanted to be part of the network of practitioners helping people. So I ditched my corporate job and I studied to become a certified sex and relationship practitioner and somatic therapist.

I've been working in private practice for eight years, and every day I support individuals, couples and groups to become more aware of their bodies, sex and sexuality. I do a fair bit of work outside the therapy room too. I'm the co-founder of NORMAL, a sexual wellness company. I'm also a writer and speaker, and over the years I have worked to create dozens of accessible educational courses and resources.

My job, and the intention of this book, is to create a safe space for enquiry while working through something edgy.

It's to equip you with the foundational tools for great sex and relationships, and offer information and practices that people often assume they should just know, despite most of us not being afforded the opportunity to learn. I've observed how simple yet effective tools can radically shift how my clients think and feel about sex. On many occasions I've seen this change happen in just a one-hour session. They leave knowing a fulfilling sex life is possible. It's not a quick fix and they have work to do in between sessions, but I hold the hope for them until they can hold it for themselves. The most rewarding part of my work is seeing how the client who came into my practice feeling small can leave feeling regulated, safe and with hope.

Not everyone can get into session with a practitioner and there are many barriers to accessing help for their particular concern or question. While I am not suggesting this book should be a substitute for therapy, perhaps it will provide you with a few tools that you can turn to if and when you are ready.

About the book

My approach

This book has a lot of information in it. You may have lightbulb moments as you're reading or you may feel validated by how much you already know about your own pleasure. But it's the way you experience this book that will be different from the other sex books you might have read.

The most important thing you will learn from me is: you learn by doing. Each chapter ends with a Practice and Play section, in which I invite you to put what we've discussed into practice. These exercises are informed by top-down and bottom-up therapeutic approaches, which might sound like therapy speak, but let me assure you, they are fundamentally very practical. Top-down means starting with the mind to get into the body, and bottom-up starts with the body to work with the mind. When we're having sex, we're not just floating minds and we're also not bodies free from thought. We've got to bring awareness to the whole of us.

Top-down therapy starts with how we are thinking: noticing how we are speaking to ourselves and others, both internally and externally, which emotions we are focused on and how we interpret information. Top-down can also refer to a lot of the traditional therapy modalities, which use talk therapy in order to observe and manage our thoughts.

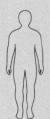 Bottom-up is often referred to as somatic therapy, and essentially refers to bringing awareness to the body. A lot of information is received and experienced in our bodies; when you feel nervous you may feel butterflies in your stomach, when you're turned on you may feel heat and sensitivity in your genitals. Sex and pleasure are all about bringing awareness to the body, whether that means processing a not-so-great experience, or practising to stay present and mindful so that you feel more pleasure. Bottom-up approaches are also essential when working with trauma, particularly in relation to our fight, flight, freeze or fawn responses. Sometimes we can't think our way out of feeling bad and we can't think our way into feeling good. Instead, we need to address what's going on in the body.

The foundations

I've done my best to cover a lot, but sex is fucking huge. The book is split into three sections: Solo Pleasure, which focuses on all the foundational tools you can explore on your own; Pleasure Together, which looks at how to create and maintain fulfilling sex and relationships with others; and Exploring Pleasure, which encourages you to continue exploring what intrigues you.

While I think it'll be most useful to move through the book from start to finish, if you're like me, you may have a nostalgic urge to flip to the most salacious chapter and metaphorically tear the textured edge of the sealed section. Move through the book however you like. It's your process. But even if you think a chapter isn't for you, I suggest staying with it: read it, integrate the learning, do the activity. Some of our most profound insights come when we least expect them.

Language

In this book, you will see terms like people with penises/vulvas, cis women and trans men. Whether you're new to this language or it's a pretty standard part of your vernacular, language is extremely important. My education and teaching is inclusive; everybody is welcome, invited and accepted. I am always really curious about an individual's experience of gender, and I intend to leave my own assumptions at the door. The language

in this book will reflect my curiosity, care and respect for others. I believe gender is a social construct; it varies from society to society and can change over time. Sexuality is also not fixed nor binary; it is individual. Not all people with penises who have sex with people with penises are gay men. The same goes for people with vulvas who have sex with people with penises; this does not necessarily mean they're straight. They may be queer, bi, pansexual, heterosexual, trans, non-binary and so on. There's an extensive list of these terms in the glossary at the end of the book.

You don't need to be an expert in gender identity to read this book. Just remember that you know more about your sexuality and gender than anyone else. And if you're still exploring it – well, perhaps these pages will give you the space to do so.

When I use the term 'partner', I'm not just describing people in long-term relationships. I'm using it to describe the other person in your sexual experience, whether casual or long-term. This book is for everyone, regardless of their relationship style.

I also swear a lot in this book. I love swearing, I think it's fun, and funny, and hot. I don't believe in policing bodies, expressions or profanities. When we can liberate ourselves from conservative thinking and language, we get closer to ourselves and further away from what is expected from us and what we think we should be doing.

Stories

I've included examples from clients I've worked with either in session or workshops over the years, as well as fantasies that were submitted anonymously to be a part of this book. All names and identifiable features have been changed. Some examples are a combination of people and stories.

Bias

I am a cis, white, able-bodied, educated, queer woman. While I have worked to diversify my training, supervisions and learning experiences to ensure I can support all people with nuance and care, I want to acknowledge that I approach this work with the privilege of moving through the world with these identities. I chose to study somatic sexology and to learn at the Institute of Somatic Sexology rather than to go back to university so that I would have access

to diverse and new ways of thinking, and to ensure I could learn from practitioners who worked outside a purely academic scene. Where and how I've studied is part of my process in decolonising pleasure, but this book is informed by my experiences in life and work and I want to acknowledge the limitations that may bring.

Sex is changing

The way we understand and experience sex is changing. More people are curious, and they're reclaiming and expressing themselves in ways that go beyond the traditional binary. It is very likely that there will be a time when some of the information and approaches I offer in this book have changed. It's likely that I will also change the way I think, speak or feel about elements in this book too. This makes me feel both nervous and hopeful. Change is a process. It is exciting, thrilling and sometimes scary. And wherever we are in the future of sex, I'll forever be learning myself. I'll be thick in that process of change with you.

My hope for you

I hope this book creates the space for you to enquire, explore and learn more about pleasure so you feel equipped to apply these learnings to real-life experiences. I hope it normalises discussion around sex and pleasure, and allows you to work through anything that's getting in the way between you and the sex life you want. There are a lot of answers, and I also ask a lot of questions. But you won't learn about pleasure by reading this book alone. Research consistently proves that it is the clients who apply the practices outside of session who notice the change they want. You're not expected to be an expert when you start this book, but if you expect change, you have to do something about it. As I said before: you learn by doing.

I hope you can speak with others about what you've learned as a way to reflect, ease the tension of individual shame and create a culture that values collective experiences over individual expertise. The more openly we can speak about sex, pleasure and bodies, the more we can normalise and celebrate human sexuality.

Our world favours binaries: normal or abnormal, right or wrong, kinky or vanilla, prude or slut, feminine or masculine. In my work, and in this book, I hope to move beyond these binaries. While I hope this book equips you with the knowledge to discover what you like and even who you are as a sexual person, there is not one right way to have sex or to be sexual. I hope it offers you the tools and ideas you need to go away and explore for yourself.

My professional experience and training gives me a degree of insight into human sexuality. But I am not and could never be an expert on your body. Only you can truly know yourself. I am completely non-attached to fixing people, because you, my friend, are not broken. We've just been let down by a society and culture that's never given us the tools and space to learn.

Before you begin reading, I invite you to do something that brings you immense pleasure – be it a type of touch, an experience, a particular food or drink, an orgasm. I did the same every time I sat down to write this book. It was written with pleasure, and its only intention is to allow space for you to experience more pleasure. How you do that is entirely up to you.

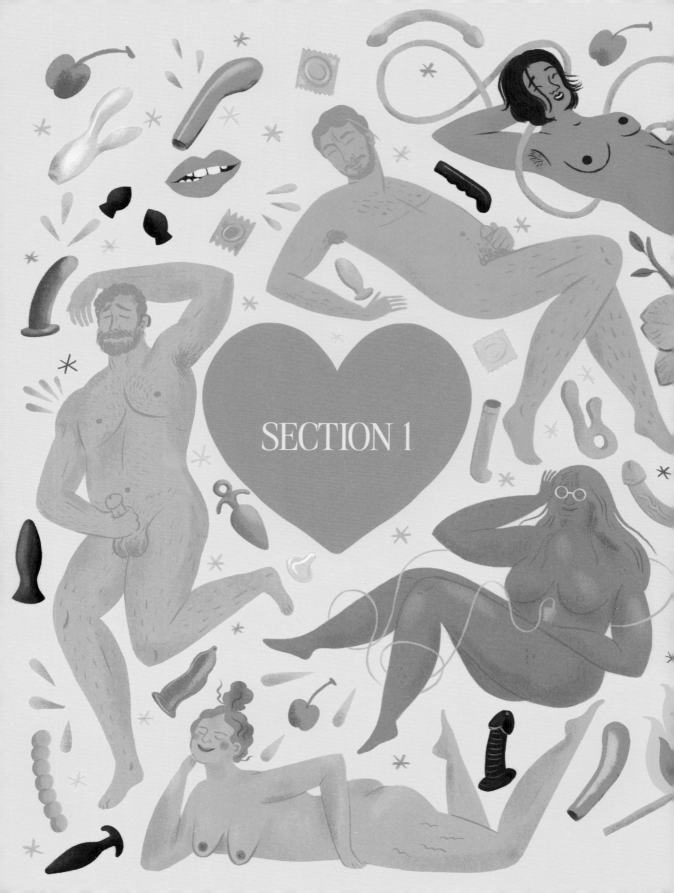

SECTION 1

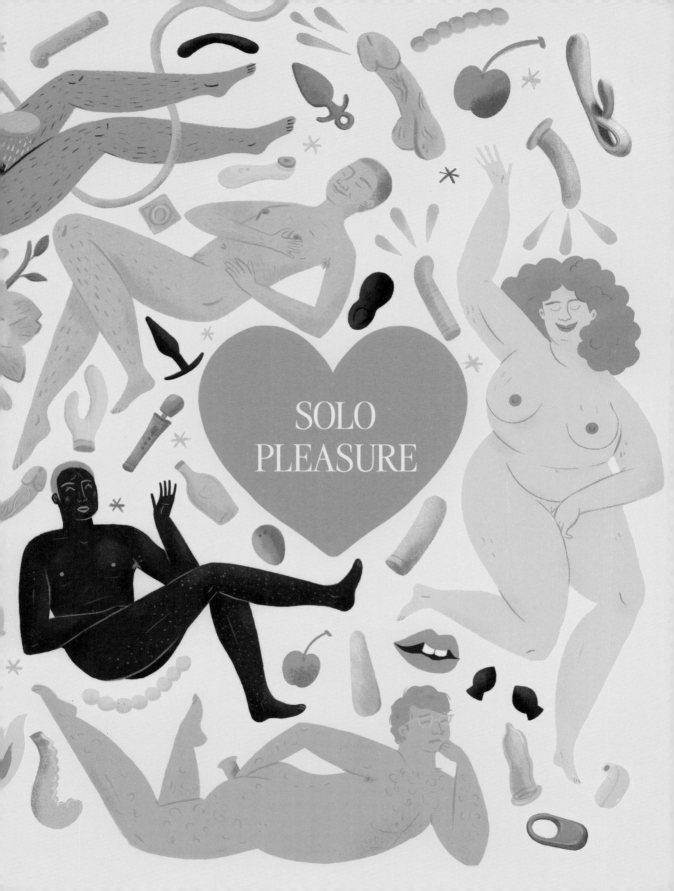

SOLO
PLEASURE

SEX, SEXUALITY AND IDENTITY

What even is sex? And what does it mean to you? What is sexual identity? How do you figure it all out? This chapter gives you the 101 on sexuality and offers some prompts to support you in defining and exploring what sexuality means to you.

Define sex. This is something even I struggle with, despite thinking, speaking and writing about it for most of my waking and sleeping moments. In many ways, this whole book is an attempt to define sex, and despite my best efforts, I still probably won't get close. In the mainstream, sex is mostly understood as the act of two (just two, folks!) naked bodies penetrating each other. But sex is a complex human experience, and means many different things to many different people, which becomes very obvious when I ask a couple to define sex – I'll get two very different answers.

So instead of seeking a single universal definition, I often find myself asking my clients, *What does a fulfilling sex life mean to you?* The answers are always surprising. Never, in the hundreds of times I've asked this question, has anyone said a fulfilling sex life means 'lots of penetration'. More often, they will mention what drives them to sex. They'll speak about pleasure, connection, exploration, orgasm, power dynamics, transcending the mundane, an expression of their identity, love, playfulness … They'll talk about the way sex makes them feel, rather than about the specific act.

In this section, as we work through the body, techniques and anatomy, this information should be seen as inspiration, rather than prescription. Techniques are important – they are our tools for feeling good, they're our foundation to build on – but more often than not, the best sex is not about the five top fingering techniques. Great sex is when we're attuned to our bodies and/or other people's bodies.

Simplistic ideas of sex can help us make sense of it – that's why sex is still mostly understood through the hetero lens of *penis in vagina*. Reducing sex to an act of naked penetration alone gives us a clear definition. We get it. Our brains really like being able to fit things into specific boxes, and sex is no different. A clear definition helps us feel normal. It may feel too revealing to admit that actually we just want to dry hump on the couch for 20 minutes or have someone suck our toes without ever taking our clothes off. But sex is changing – how we experience it, our curiosities, and what we do with our bodies or other people's bodies. Sex can be anything you want it to be. So long as everyone involved is consenting, is free to leave whenever they want, and is experiencing no unwanted pain, then it's up to you to figure out what it is that you like and want.

In theory this is freeing, but in reality it can be daunting. Many of us want a checklist of all the things sex could be so we can measure what it is to us. Instead, let's start by getting to know who you are – this can help you get closer to what you want.

WHAT IS SEXUALITY?

Sexuality is complex, and our own understanding of it can be an ever-evolving process. Sexuality is often seen and understood in binaries: gay or straight, sexual or non-sexual.

♥ 13

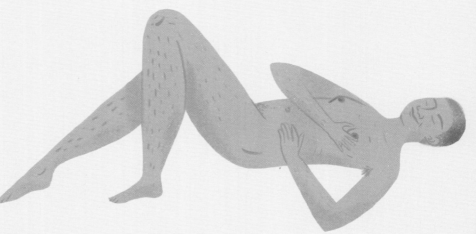

For some people, this aligns with their expression of themselves – but it's not the only way to experience sexuality. Binaries can help us make sense of who we are and how we fit in with people, cultures or ideas; they can also limit us. Human sexuality is complex. It's not just about who we want to have sex with – it can be about our sexual orientation, attraction, desires and behaviours. It is a meaningful part of our human experience and plays a key role in how we form sexual and non-sexual relationships, how we express affection and how we experience pleasure.

Labels can be validating for some and limiting for others, and sometimes they are the stepping stone to really figuring out who we are, what we want and what we're into. Whoever you are or wherever you're at right now, there's so much to sexuality, often so much humanness and depth of experience, that it can't neatly fit into one word.

Let's look at a few key components.

✳ Sexual orientation: This often refers to our emotional, romantic and/or sexual attraction to a specific gender or person, but it can also be about asexuality, not wanting to have sex. Sexual orientation is a natural and intrinsic aspect of a person's identity.

✳ Gender identity: Gender identity relates to a person's internal sense of their own gender, which may or may not align with the sex they were assigned at birth. Gender identity is distinct from biological sex, which is determined by physical characteristics. It is a fundamental aspect of an individual's self-identity and understanding of who they are. Gender identity is not strictly tied to biological or physical characteristics and can go way beyond the binary of gender being male and female. We don't need to understand someone's identity to respect and affirm their gender, and using their name and pronouns is a crucial aspect of supporting their gender identity.

✳ Sexual expression: Sexual expression refers to the way we express ourselves sexually. This can include how we behave, our preferences and our practices. Our sexual expression can be about how we move our bodies, how we flirt, what we do with others. It can also be a choice around how we dress or present ourselves.

✳ Romantic attraction: Beyond sexual attraction, we may also experience romantic attraction, which involves emotional connections, affection and love. These attractions can be heteroromantic, homoromantic, biromantic or aromantic.

When I say that understanding our sexuality is an ever-evolving process, I want to emphasise the word *process*. Knowing ourselves is really useful, but it can be rigid. I am not interested in knowing myself completely – I am more interested in having an awareness of who I am, while also recognising that will probably change. I hope we can all feel a sense of ease in knowing we will constantly learn, change and experience our bodies and sex in new ways throughout life. We are not fixed; we are always in a process of change.

WHAT DO CIS AND TRANS MEAN?

People with a gender identity that matches the sex they were assigned at birth are often described as cisgender, which we can also shorten to cis. For example, when I was born, the nurse saw I had a vulva and told my parents, 'It's a girl!' I identify as a woman; therefore, I'm a cis woman. Those whose gender identity differs from the sex that was presumed at birth may call themselves transgender, or trans for short. There's no one way to be trans; it is an umbrella term that covers a large range of genders, such as non-binary, trans masc, trans femme, genderqueer, genderfluid, a Sistergirl or Brotherboy, or it could be literally anything else they want for themselves. Their experience of gender may not sit within the confines of the male–female binary. Gender identity is deeply personal, and may be experienced in numerous ways, such as the way someone chooses to dress, their pronouns and their choice of gender-related terminology.

HOW DO I KNOW IF I'M GAY/STRAIGHT/BI/ TRANS...?

If you google this question, you'll get a completely different answer from the one I'm about to give you. I'm not going to test you or map out your sexual history in order to label you gay or straight for the rest of eternity. The only person who can decide who you are is *you*. Figuring out your sexuality can be complicated, and there is no right way to do so. Most of us have grown up thinking the default is straight, until you realise it's not, and then you come out to every single person you've ever met (which is certainly a liberating part of the process for some, but of course, not for everyone).

Nothing makes you LGBTQIA+. It is actually pretty harmful to ask, 'What made you gay?', as the question assumes that being straight is the default and that heterosexuality is normal and expected. But if you're gay, there's a heteronormative expectation to track, trace and 'reveal' cornerstones of your queer awakening that have turned you, that have made you something different from the mainstream. If we're asking what made you gay, we also need to be asking what made you straight.

Some people may learn about their sexuality after an intense and undeniable crush, watching a movie and feeling their fanny flutter, waking up from a wet dream about someone, or through the recurring fantasies they wank to, their favourite porn scene or even the string of relationships they've had. But these things also don't necessarily prove your sexual orientation. There's no one way or right way to figure it out; often it comes down to exploration, and affording yourself the space to be clunky and vulnerable while you explore. I know many of you might wish I would wave my magic sex wand and reveal the answer, but while it might be easier that way, it would also strip you of your agency and autonomy and, frankly, the joy of discovering it for yourself.

Everything is always changing, and that includes us. Sexuality can change too; it is fluid. Some people will strongly identify as one sexuality their whole life and others will change – it's all normal. If or when your sexuality evolves, it doesn't mean you're confused or late to the party. No two people are the same – and honestly, thank fuck for that. It'd be really boring if we were. If you're curious and not sure where to begin, it may be useful to start by exploring certain sexualities. Do your research and observe how your body responds. What feels like it closely speaks to your experience? And you don't have to do it on your own. Finding your community is so valuable, be it online or in person, at a party or a book club. Try to connect with supportive, accepting people, whether they're a bestie, family member or professional.

My queer clients will often ask, 'Am I gay enough?' – a question I've also taken to my own therapy sessions. How will people read me if I don't have a mullet? How will I fit within my community and show them that I, too, am very gay? And at the same time, while I'm trying to fit in, how do I get closer to creating my own sense of what it means to be queer?

I often think about how bell hooks, American author, theorist, educator and social critic, spoke about queerness. She thinks about '"being queer" not as being about who you're having sex with – that can be a dimension of it – but "queer" as being about the self that is at odds with everything around it and it has to invent and create and find a place to speak and to thrive and to live'.

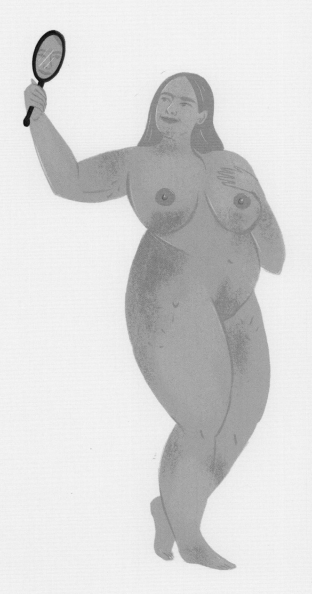

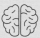 ## Sexual curiosity and attraction

Because sexuality is individual and personal, solo enquiry into what it actually means for us is always useful. Some people may start their enquiry in their teens, but I've had plenty of clients who start in their sixties. You're never too late to the game – after all, it is a lifelong process. Wherever you're at, consider the following (not so simple) questions:

✳ Who am I?

✳ Who/what am I attracted to (including gender, personality, values, genitals, bodies ...)?

✳ Who was the last person who caught my eye and made me feel something (aroused, excited, nervous)?

✳ If I could experience my sexuality as a blob rather than a spectrum, what would be in this blob?

✳ What am I curious about?

✳ What do I know I never want to try?

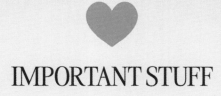

IMPORTANT STUFF

✳ Only you decide your sexuality.

✳ You cannot assume you know someone's sexuality based on the way they dress or speak, what they do for work, who they date or who they've had sex with.

✳ Sexuality is unique, complex and ever evolving.

✳ Nothing 'makes' you LGBTQIA+. If we're asking what makes you gay, we also need to be asking what makes you straight.

✳ You don't have to come out to anyone if you don't want to.

✳ If someone is homophobic, that's their issue, not yours. You are not wrong. The only thing morally wrong here is bigotry.

✳ Everyone has always had a 'first' – it's never too late.

✳ Community is essential, healing and validating. Create and connect with people who help you feel seen and safe.

✳ Seek support when and if you need. There are so many resources, organisations and practitioners out there who can support you.

FEELING PRESENT

Feeling distracted, anxious or unable
to relax during sex is really common.
This chapter covers some essential
techniques to feel more present,
connected and regulated during sex.

Most people will be familiar with this feeling. You're having
sex or masturbating, and you really want to be present
and connected to your body – but your mind is wandering.
You're thinking about your never-ending to-do list, or that
thing you forgot to do at work, or whether your neighbours
can hear you, or how you look from that angle, or if you
smell or taste okay, or why you're taking so long to cum,
or that you need to call your mum back … then wtf why am
I thinking about my mum?

Most people want to get out of their heads and into their
bodies, but it's virtually impossible to shut our brains off
completely. When we're having sex, we're not just a body
that's completely free from thinking and feeling. Instead of
'getting out of your head', it's far more useful to build a mind
and body connection.

I find a lot of my clients feel overwhelmed when they try to 'shut off' their thoughts. This can be hard, and that's okay – we want your brain to think! What's going on in your mind has a direct impact on your sexual experience – and sometimes it can even be used to energise experiences. Thoughts can turn you on.

Eastern practices of mindfulness have been around for centuries, but it's only since neurological research has begun to prove the benefits of mindfulness on our overall health and wellbeing that the Western world has jumped on board. At risk of getting a little too sex-geeky, I want to break down not only why we turn to mindfulness as the basis of so many therapeutic approaches but also how it directly relates to sex.

When practised regularly, mindfulness can lead to changes in brain structure and function that enhance the capacity to experience pleasure. It can reduce the intrusion of challenging emotions, thoughts and distractions, increase sensory awareness and promote a more positive emotional state, all of which support a heightened experience of pleasure. The neuroscience of mindfulness shows its potential to rewire the brain in ways that can improve someone's overall sense of wellbeing and enjoyment.

BODY AWARENESS

Mindfulness practices are foundational in addressing many of the sexual concerns I work with. When I ask people, 'What are you noticing in your body?' – even if they don't know what they're feeling – their first response is often to cry. For possibly the first time, they have brought awareness to how they feel – tense, hopeless, lost, broken – and it's all experienced physically. But not everyone is on board with it straight away. Clients will often answer, 'I don't know', 'What do you mean?', 'Why is this relevant?' It's learning a new way into your body, and that can feel clunky at first. It takes time and practice to build the connection.

One of my clients once said, 'Why do you keep asking me what I'm noticing in my body? It's really annoying.' She was seeing me because she'd never had an orgasm and felt really disconnected from her body. She hated when sexual partners tried desperately to be the first to make her cum, cure her, fix her problem. At that moment, I was a threat to her. I was just another person asking for information about her body – information she was unable to give. This is such a common response.

It's a great question, though – why did I want to know what she was feeling in her body? What's the usefulness of that? Our bodies can often be a vast source of information about how we're feeling. Sometimes we can't think our way in or out of a thought spiral, or think our way back to sex. Instead, sometimes we need to feel our way through. I ask these questions so that people can practise bringing more attention to what they're noticing outside of a sexual context, so that it's a bit easier in a sexual context.

SEX AND STRESS

You're a human, so you've probably felt stress before. Stress can have a huge impact on how you're feeling in your own body, but also on how you're feeling in your relationships. Stress around sex and relationships may also be your very reason for reading this book. It's worth noting that if you're really struggling at the moment, I strongly recommend seeing a specialist.

When you're stressed, your body goes through a series of changes in order to keep you safe – aka your fight, flight, freeze, fawn response. This is your body's natural reaction to danger; it is an automatic reaction that is designed to keep us alive. That's ideal if we're being chased by a sabre-toothed tiger, but probably not essential in every moment of our day.

When we're operating in a state of chronic stress, we may respond to certain triggers by choosing to *fight* with our words or actions, *flight* to get out of there, *freeze* to pause to assess the next move, or *fawn* to appease or please the aggressor by minimising or avoiding the threat.

Window of tolerance

Dr Dan Siegel coined this term to describe the state of being in which a person feels grounded, regulated and safe. Within the window of tolerance, people feel they can move throughout the world with ease. They can observe, process and respond to triggers or stimuli without being sent into survival mode. They're also able to connect and feel present in new experiences.

Staying in this window is really tricky for anyone living with trauma or anxiety, or for those who are chronically stressed.

A trigger (that may seem insignificant to someone else) can push them outside their window of tolerance, into either hyper-arousal or hypo-arousal.

Hyper-arousal is a fight/flight response – i.e. perceiving danger, you prepare to fight or get out of there to keep yourself safe. This can mean constantly scanning your environment, having racing thoughts, and feeling your heart pumping faster. Hypo-arousal, on the other hand, is the freeze response. Your systems shut down, you find it hard to formulate sentences, stay present or communicate, and you may feel distant or disassociate.

Many people are operating in these states on a daily basis – at work, at home, in their relationships or even when thinking about sex. This affects us both physically and emotionally. When I show the window of tolerance to clients, they often have a lightbulb moment, and can suddenly understand that there's nothing wrong with them. They're not too much, they're not broken; it's just that the way they're responding to a stimulus is based on past experiences.

When you're in survival mode, it can be hard to bring sex to the front of your mind or consider it a priority – after all, your body and nervous system are essentially focusing on keeping you alive, even if cognitively you know there's no real life-threatening danger. All of this can impact your mood and desire, your energy or capacity to connect with your partner, and your ability to feel pleasure and sensation. Because this is so common, I teach stress management, self-regulation and mindfulness practices to the majority of my clients to help them get into that window of tolerance to feel more regulated.

Let's give it a go.

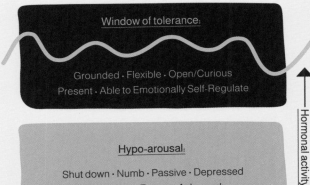

Hyper-arousal:

High energy · Anxious · Angry · Overwhelmed
Hypervigilant · Responding with fight/flight · Chaotic

Window of tolerance:

Grounded · Flexible · Open/Curious
Present · Able to Emotionally Self-Regulate

Hypo-arousal:

Shut down · Numb · Passive · Depressed
Withdrawn · Frozen · Ashamed

Hormonal activity

Time

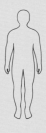

Building body awareness

Mindfulness is a skill. It's not something you need to be 'good at', but often it is something that takes practice. Ask yourself:

✳ What am I noticing in my body right now?

✳ What is my body trying to tell me?

✳ How is this physically showing up in my body?

✳ What can I do for my body right now?

By building awareness of how your body is feeling outside of a sexual context, it will be less challenging to be aware of your body during sex. As an extension, we want to start finding a way to regulate that feeling – but not necessarily change it or make it go away entirely.

Then feel into the question: 'What's between me and feeling fine? Not exceptional, just fine. Is there anything I can do to feel just fine? Is it three deep breaths? A moment with your feet on some grass? A big cuddle from a loved one? Moving to music?'

Ask yourself this whenever you feel spun out, stressed or overwhelmed.

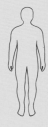

Simple practice to self-regulate

Here's a two-part process to find a way into your window of tolerance. This can help you feel regulated, grounded and safe.

Awareness

Bring awareness to any moments when you feel like you're outside of your window of tolerance. Notice what that feels like. It may even be worth naming it: 'I notice I'm feeling X.'

Regulation

What can you do to regulate your body? Consider breath, movement, sound, touch, placement of awareness, fast-paced movement like running on the spot, soothing touch or grounding practices.

Tools for staying present outside of a sexual context

Breathe in

Hold

Box breathing

Hold

Breathe out

✳ **Ground yourself.** Stand, sit, or lie in a position that supports you in feeling grounded. Feel for a sense of gravity that is allowing you to be in that space. Lengthen your exhale.

✳ **Observe.** Look around the room and name everything you see for one minute.

✳ **Breathe.** Try breathing in the shape of a box (see the diagram above) for four equal counts. Breathe in for four, hold for four, out for four, hold for four. Do this for a few rounds.

✳ **Self-soothe with touch.** Placing one hand on your chest and one on your lower stomach may feel calming, as you can also feel for your breath.

✳ **Move to a rhythm.** Sway from side to side or bounce a ball.

✳ **Listen to a meditation.** Let it guide you.

✳ **5, 4, 3, 2, 1.** Name five things you can see, four things you can feel, three things you can hear, two things you can smell and one thing you can taste.

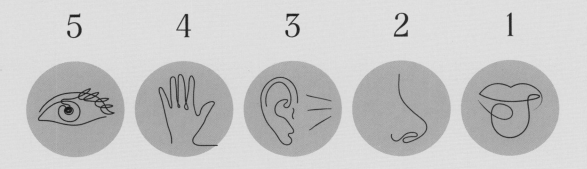

5   4   3   2   1

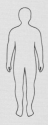

Practising staying present during a sexual context

Try one of these at a time. It may be useful once, and you may need to try something different next time.

✳ Bring your awareness to the sensation in your body and what feels good or pleasurable in this moment.

✳ Name it. This could be as simple as: 'I'm noticing I'm/you're distracted. Can we take a moment to reconnect?'

✳ Pause. Slow things down and take a moment to bring your awareness back to your body.

✳ Mobilise. If you're feeling stuck, frozen or disassociated, try mobilising your body. Stand up, shake, move, go to the bathroom or splash cold water on your face.

✳ Ask for space while you regulate.

✳ Connect with yourself or others. Ask for a specific type of touch like a hug or a kiss.

This isn't something that will change instantly. If you're spending most of your day disconnected from your body, you won't magically be able to be mindful during sex. At times this can feel tough to handle on your own – because our mental state can impact our whole lives, not just our sex lives. Dealing with this is a gradual process, and I recommend seeing a specialist if it doesn't start to feel more manageable after working on it yourself. This support could involve sessions with a practitioner in a modality that's right for you, mindfulness, stress management, lifestyle changes like rest, yummy food and exercise, and learning how to lean on your social network can all be really useful.

IMPORTANT STUFF

✳ If you're not feeling present during sex, know that you're not alone. This is SO human. There will be moments throughout every sexual experience where you're distracted or your mind wanders. This isn't necessarily a bad thing, but in order to feel more pleasure and sensation, it'll be useful to practise bringing your awareness back to the present moment.

✳ We can talk about being more mindful all day, but you will learn by doing. Grounding practices, guided meditation, breathwork and mindful masturbation can all be useful in helping you stay present.

✳ You'll need to practise being present outside of a sexual context regularly, like multiple times a week. This will support you in feeling more present during sex.

SEXUAL CONFIDENCE

This chapter covers body image and sexual confidence. Learn about the common blockages and issues affecting sexual confidence, and explore techniques for rewiring unhelpful beliefs, communicating your needs and exploring what turns you on (and off).

Have you ever felt uncomfortable being naked, felt nervous about trying something new, struggled to voice your desires or felt undeserving of pleasure because of your appearance? At the core, you may be struggling with low sexual confidence, which statistics show is one of the most common sexual concerns. You're not alone, and there's a lot you can do.

Sexual confidence is built by doing, because sex is a skill. And like any skill, the more we do it, the more comfortable, confident and capable we feel. Of course, in reality it's not that simple. For those who feel unwilling, nervous or lacking in confidence, we need to look at what's getting in the way. These aren't small things. We need to understand the context, how we think, how we feel and the things we do.

 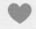

LET'S JUMP IN

Sexual confidence can affect all aspects of life, and directly impacts how we feel during sex and in our relationships. It's not just something that comes up in the few minutes you're having sex. It can be on your mind throughout the day; it can show up in the way you avert your gaze from the attractive person in the bar, or it may prevent you from ever touching your partner due to the fear that the touch may give your partner the wrong idea.

Sexual confidence will look and feel different for everyone. For some, it's being able to ask someone out on a date; for others, it's knowing what to offer or ask for during sex. There's not one single definition, but I notice a few recurrent themes with my clients. Sexual confidence is when:

✳ You feel comfortable in your own body.

✳ You have an awareness of your wants, needs and desires.

✳ You're comfortable communicating or advocating for your body.

✳ You feel safe and grounded.

✳ You have tools to regulate your nervous system back to a space of presence.

✳ You feel comfortable when you look in the mirror.

✳ You speak kindly and compassionately to your body.

✳ You value your body for its function and capacity to experience pleasure.

✳ You feel worthy and deserving of pleasure.

✳ You enjoy, value and prioritise sex.

✳ You approach sex with playfulness and curiosity.

✳ You see sex as an experience, not a performance.

I want all of this for everyone, and it is possible. But it's not as simple as repeating the mantra 'I am hot', and it's definitely not something that can be 'fixed' by signing up for the *six-week bangin' beach bod challenge*.

WHERE DOES LOW CONFIDENCE COME FROM?

Have you ever considered that perhaps it's not just on you? Our confidence and self-image are constantly bombarded with damaging messages from influences such as the media, cultural ideals, sexism, capitalism, ableism – all the 'isms' – religion, a lack of diversity and limited education.

In order to build confidence, we need to liberate ourselves from these systems. You might do all this incredible work in therapy, at home, in the choices you make and the way you speak to yourself, but you still have to exist within these oppressive systems. I'm pointing this out not to disempower you, but to acknowledge that our confidence is connected to our overall identity, the way we view ourselves within the world and the systems that surround us. Please keep this in mind as we work through this chapter.

Sometimes the most liberating thing we can do is to say fuck you to these systems, to collectively masturbate at 3 pm, to reject the idea that we are unworthy of pleasure until we earn it. Pleasure is political, pleasure is radical, pleasure is resistance against systems that oppress us. As the pioneering pleasure activist Adrienne Maree Brown says, 'Pleasure is a measure of freedom.'

QUESTIONS TO ASK OURSELVES

The following questions can help identify and confront various assumptions, beliefs or unhelpful thoughts you might hold towards yourself. You can then counteract these thought patterns by presenting evidence that is more neutral and 'fair', helping you to reframe or challenge these ideas.

* What is the assumption I would like to adjust?

* Where might this assumption have come from? Why may it still be here?

* What impact does this assumption have on my life?

* What impact does this assumption have on my relationship with my body or sex?

* In what ways is this assumption unreasonable, unrealistic or unhelpful?

* What is an alternative assumption that is more balanced and flexible?

* What can I do to put this assumption into practice on a daily basis?

It's not all on you. Again, fuck the system, not you. Or fuck yourself *and* the system – now that's activism!

HOW WE THINK ABOUT BODY CONFIDENCE

When we think about body confidence, there are two approaches that float around: body positivity and body neutrality.

Body positivity

As we know it today, body positivity is a celebration of all bodies that promotes acceptance regardless of shape, colour, size, gender, sexuality or ability. It wants us to believe all bodies are beautiful, worthy and deserving of love and pleasure. And I'm all in for that part! Celebrating bodies is an important part of sexual confidence.

Body positivity started as a social movement led by fat liberation activists in the late sixties. Radical fat activism was spearheaded by ethnic minority women who protested against structural discrimination and oppression, particularly from unrealistic fashion and beauty standards capitalising on communities to make them feel inadequate.

However, the growing popularity of the term 'body positive' has also seen the advent of performative activism, with already thin people pushing out their tummies on Instagram, as well as queer and disabled bodies, who were foundational in the emergence of body positivity, being excluded from the movement.

Writer Amanda Mull argued in her article 'Body positivity is a scam' that by failing to acknowledge body positivity's radical past, the current movement ignores structural systems of oppression, such as racism, sexism, ableism and homophobia, that lead to negative body image. Now, what we're seeing is an obsession with feeling shit hot all the time. This focus has led to toxic positivity, which can deny the reality or difficulties people face, adding more pressure and psychological stress. We slap shame on shame – *Oh, you don't feel good in your body? That's really bad! Here, buy some rose-scented cream and run yourself a bath.*

Body neutrality

Many have moved away from body positivity towards neutrality, which sits somewhere between body negativity and body positivity. Body neutrality means you don't loathe *or* love your body – you accept and respect it for its functions and what it can do, rather than what it looks like. Body neutrality acknowledges that happiness, joy and pleasure shouldn't be reliant on how your body looks, that we are complex beings with thoughts, feelings and emotions. I find body neutrality to be pretty useful in session, especially when it comes to sexual pleasure and function. You don't need to be obsessed with the way your stomach looks in order to cum. There's a lot of pleasure and sensation to be experienced even in the parts of your body you dislike the most. Neutrality, however, doesn't celebrate the body, which for many is an important part of feeling sexually confident.

Body acceptance

I interviewed my friend Demon Derriere, a fat activist, model and burlesque dancer, and they said they suspected body neutrality was thought up by a thin white woman. They said that people with white, cis, thin, abled bodies are afforded the space to be neutral about their bodies. As an alternative, Demon offered body acceptance as a tool to firmly view your body as good enough, seeing social and cultural beauty standards as separate and creating your own standards for yourself.

EXAMINE, CHALLENGE, REFRAME

I've outlined these approaches in order to illustrate the tools available to you at any given moment. Sometimes things are useful, sometimes they're not. And if body neutrality or body positivity is particularly useful for you, then stick with it. There are benefits and limitations in all of it. We're constantly sifting through conflicting messages. We're bombarded with body-focused messaging in our capitalist society, which profits from shame and taboo around the body, paired with the expectation that in this emerging sexual revolution, we should be DTF at the drop of a hat. Finding our own experience among all this is confusing.

There's also a pretty valid argument that these approaches are far too simplistic. A lot of my clients are like, 'Gimme the science!' I've certainly been in that camp too. I mean, come on – I'm expected to repeat 'I'm beautiful' in the mirror every day and believe it when I have trolls on social media saying I look like 'budget Keira Knightley' or commenting with vomit emojis on my posts? That said, it's really useful to examine the way we speak to our bodies on a regular basis.

Negativity bias is something we are all susceptible to. It's the experience of being drawn to the negative rather than the positive information, outcome, news or feedback around us. We're constantly scanning our environment, assessing potential threats or danger. And sometimes the threat we identify can be the way we look. Like catching your reflection in a window on your way to work, noticing a bloated belly or a pimple on your chin and hearing a critical thought loop start up, wiping out the other ways you might have felt about your body during the rest of the week.

Confirmation bias, on the other hand, is our tendency to scan our environment and 'cherry pick' bits of information that confirm what we already believe. This, again, is a pretty useful resource we've developed over time to keep us 'safe'. However, it is unhelpful when our core beliefs or narratives are harsh towards ourselves.

To rewire this thinking, many turn to cognitive behavioural therapy (CBT), a top-down cognitive reframing that suggests our emotions, thoughts, behaviour and body sensations are all linked, and that what we do and what we

think will affect the way we feel. I'll give you an example. One of my clients had never had sex, even though they'd had many opportunities with people and they really, really wanted to have sex. They felt increasingly nervous about their first time. By the time it came to sex, they would shut things down and cut off all communication. This made them feel even more inexperienced, unloved and hopeless, and they started to think there was no point in dating at all, as it was bound to be a stressful experience.

Some common CBT strategies or 'tools' they could use would be to challenge the negative thoughts with more neutral or positive thoughts, finding more evidence for things that are based in 'reality' or rational thought. They could reframe a thought into something more 'fair', neutral or positive towards themselves. Over time, this redirection of thought could lead to a more nuanced and neutral thought process, which may also ease the physiological symptoms that negative thought patterns were having on their overall health and body.

I'll be honest, I'm not all in for CBT. I think it's useful when considered as part of a larger toolkit, but a valid criticism is that it's too simplistic in its approach. It is issue-centred and problem-focused and places all responsibility on the individual to fix their 'irrational' thoughts so that they can get back to being a 'normal' member of society and straight back to work. Philosophically, I can't get behind the power sitting with mainstream ideology of irrational thinking, as it doesn't consider the context in which the individual exists: the chaos, connection, lived experience, community, culture, emotions. CBT also does not take into account how the body is feeling in order to understand the trigger that leads to feeling shit in that moment.

I asked my sex-avoidant client, 'What happens in your body when you think you might have sex with someone new?' They told me their body tenses up, shoulders tight to their ears, and they feel like they are frozen, which makes them want to run away. Not a sexy feeling at all. I asked them, 'What is your body telling you at that moment, and what is it that you need in order to come back to feeling safe and confident?' At the core, they were terrified they would embarrass themselves, and felt that they needed to perform for their new sexual partners in order to feel loved. They placed so much expectation on being the best sexual partner, that they never gave themself the opportunity to learn.

THE LEARNING EDGE

In order to support this client, I needed to walk with them to their learning edge. The learning edge is where change happens. It feels clunky, awkward and uncomfortable, because you're doing things differently. The edge is doing the thing you know is useful, but for whatever reason it hasn't felt possible. It is not about pushing boundaries or going beyond what feels safe, but it's also not about staying in the 'known' and doing what you're already doing.

My client needed to find their edge to prove to themself that they were able to do something new and that they could *survive it* (which they did). We held the goal of feeling confident but broke it down into smaller, more accessible, more achievable milestones.

For them, this started by letting new sexual partners know how far they wanted to go: kissing with clothes off felt edgy enough. This in itself was a confidence-building exercise – voicing the desire 'I just want to kiss' made them feel powerful and assured. They were surprised that every single new sexual partner was equally on board. No one wanted to go further, as they felt a little nervous too. Then my client started telling sexual partners, 'I want to learn about your body and how you like to be touched, what you like and don't like. Can you be really descriptive so I can make sure I'm doing things that feel good for you?'

They dropped the pressure of needing to be an expert and started asking questions instead. They came back to session and said that even though they were practising, it was some of the hottest experiences they'd ever had. They felt connected to their own body and to the other person's. They were also getting all the information they needed, and their confidence grew, because the experience of it proved they were a good lover. They integrated what Peggy Kleinplatz famously said – great lovers aren't born, they're made.

THE EMOTIONAL LANDSCAPE OF CONFIDENCE

Our emotional experiences are directly related to how we feel about our bodies and sex, and they can often get in the way of our confidence. Even during casual sex, you're still going to feel emotions – it may not be love, but it could be lust, excitement, disgust, shame. Our emotions act as

messages. They tell us if something feels safe, sexy or even scary. Often when we're struggling with confidence, something unknown may feel scary, uncomfortable or unsafe, so it's tempting to tap out or disconnect.

We can build confidence by trusting that we'll be able to acknowledge how we feel, and recognising a need based on that. And one way of doing that is to use the feelings wheel (on the next page), developed by Dr Gloria Willcox. It can help you get a little closer to identifying your emotion and how it feels for you.

The wheel is divided into three sections: **primary emotions**, a fundamental or general sense of how we're feeling; **secondary emotions**, which show that emotions are nuanced and rarely singular and that we can experience a complex blend of feelings at once; and **tertiary emotions**, the subtle differences that make all our emotional responses feel different. I find this wheel offers useful information, giving us greater awareness of how we feel, which helps us understand certain triggers, and what we may need to regulate these responses.

The Feelings Wheel, developed by Dr Gloria Willcox

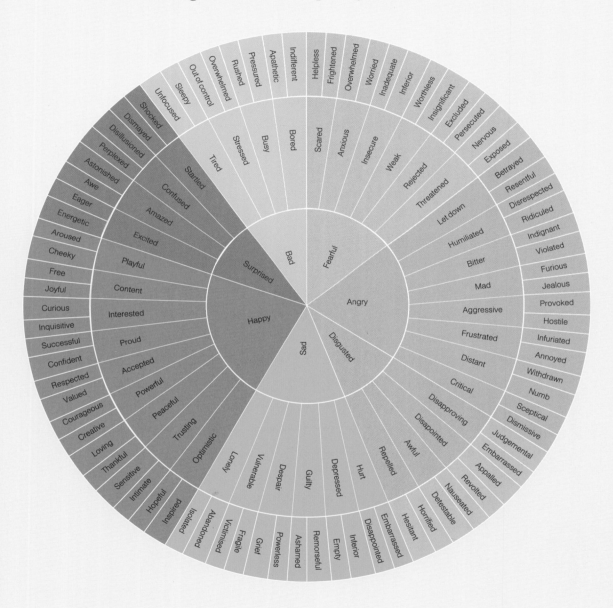

It's still sometimes tricky to identify what we are feeling, even with a guide like this. So again, we turn to the body. Emotions are felt in the body. The emotional system in our brain sends signals to help us respond to a stimulus, person or context, and different emotions activate different body parts. *I'm nervous and I feel it in my gut; I'm stressed and my chest is tight; I'm angry and I feel the tension of my jaw and fists.*

Bringing awareness to the physical sensation can help us identify the emotion we're feeling and determine what we want to do next. In 2013, Lauri Nummenmaa and others conducted a study in which participants drew maps of body locations where they feel specific emotions (see illustration below). Hot colours show regions that people say are stimulated during the emotion. Cool colours indicate deactivated areas. The same researchers continued this study in 2018. They found that the stronger the feeling is physically, the stronger it will be felt in the mind. When it comes to understanding and regulating our emotional landscapes, we can't ignore our bodies. So much of our confidence is related to how we feel physically. Learning about what we feel and when we feel it is essential.

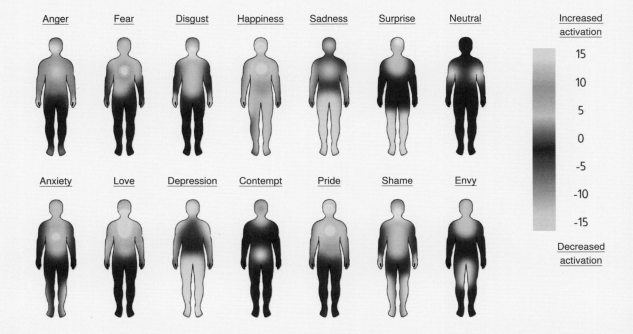

Anger | Fear | Disgust | Happiness | Sadness | Surprise | Neutral

Anxiety | Love | Depression | Contempt | Pride | Shame | Envy

Increased activation

15
10
5
0
-5
-10
-15

Decreased activation

SOMETIMES WE CAN'T THINK OUR WAY OUT OF FEELING BAD

When it comes to your own experience with body confidence, ask yourself what emotions are present, and where and how you feel them in your body. Rather than being strict and rigid with yourself, or even labelling this as good or bad information, consider how you can be flexible with these emotions instead of being paralysed by them. Instead of ignoring your emotion, compassionately enquire into where it may have surfaced from, and whether it is rational or proportionate to the situation at hand. Acknowledge how it shows up in your mind and body, and explore tools such as breath, movement, sound, touch or a shared experience with someone else to move through it.

PRACTICE AND PLAY SESSIONS

The most sexually confident people I've met are those who have had the opportunity to practise and be playful. Confidence is built when you have the space to learn and master a new skill.

The first time I cracked an egg, I was racked with fear – sure, I was only three, but I had no fucking clue. Now I crack eggs all the time and don't even think about it. In much the same way, sexual confidence is built through experience. It's a troubling and dangerous approach to assume you know what someone will want, like or need. You have to *learn* about their body. It doesn't matter if you've had sex with over a hundred different people, or if you're having sex with someone who has the same genitals as you. Everybody is different. Bad sexual partners assume; great sexual partners ask.

A practice and play session is useful regardless of the skill you're hoping to develop: massage, kissing, penetration, fingering, oral. Practice sessions do not need to end in orgasm, or even need to feel overwhelmingly arousing. Discuss the skill you want to practise (touching, kissing, anal, pegging, toys, a specific sex act, etc.), set a timer for an agreed length, ask questions, give heaps of information, check in, follow what feels good and be completely non-attached to an outcome. You're just two (or more) people seeking information while you touch and stimulate one another. Then you put those newfound skills into a play session. Here, you're curious, playful and, again, goal-free. More often than not, people will share that the best sex they've had wasn't necessarily because it ended in a big ol' orgasm; the best sex was the feeling that's co-created – bring your attention back to that.

FAT IS NOT A BAD WORD

We live in a fatphobic society that consistently tells us skinny equals sexy, healthy and successful. Many clients have shared with me that they lost all their sexual confidence after gaining weight or have never felt confident due to their shape, weight or size.

When people say 'I feel fat', what they're really trying to say is that they feel uncomfortable in their body. Fat is not a feeling; fat is a part of every human body. We can work on the feeling of being uncomfortable by using many of the tools shared in this chapter, as well as by holding compassion for feelings of shame or embarrassment, unpacking internalised fatphobia, finding community and bringing touch, pleasure and sensation to the body in an effort to build connection and embodied awareness. But we also need to challenge the notion that responsibility

rests solely on the individual. This is a collective effort. We need to examine and abolish systems of oppression that lead to fat discrimination, and the diet industries that shame, pathologise and ridicule fat bodies; we need to hold the patriarchy accountable, as well as the beauty and fashion industries, and recognise the lack of fat bodies and diversity in porn and advertising that have profited from our insecurities. There are many great practitioners who've dedicated their careers to creating tools and safe spaces; for more resources, I recommend the work of Sonalee Rashatwar and their Instagram account The Fat Sex Therapist; Tanya Koens, an Australian-based sex therapist, who offers training on the politics of pleasure; and Adrienne Maree Brown, author of *Pleasure Activism*.

It's worth noting that some people feel a great sense of shame around the word fat, while others describe themselves as fat in an effort to embrace, celebrate and reclaim the word. Fat activists may also use terms like big belly, back rolls, fupa (fatty upper pubic area), saggy tits, thick thighs, cellulite, stretch marks – these words and terms, which for so long have been used to harm, are now being

♥ 39

reclaimed in much the same way as 'slut' or 'queer' has been. If you're having sex with someone and you're unsure about how to refer to their body – ask them.

There's a lot we have to consider about specific individual experiences, particularly for fat folk with intersectional identities of being disabled, queer, trans and/or POC. My friend Demon Derriere says that when it comes to sex and relationships, 'Fat folks have experienced or are currently experiencing a different type of trauma and discrimination to everyone. We don't want to be clumped in and be told our problems or our process are the same as everyone else's.'

There are some harmful assumptions about sex and fatness that we need to put in the bin.

Myth: You'll injure your partner

Truth: This is bullshit. People get injured during sex all the time and it has nothing to do with weight or size. We all have a responsibility to start slow, not push through any unwanted pain, be aware of each other's bodies, and check in if something is uncomfortable. You're not more likely to get injured or to injure someone else because of your weight.

Myth: It's hard to find genitals

Truth: All genitals and bodies are different. Sometimes it can be challenging to stimulate the most sensitive spot on or in any body. That's why we explore different shapes and positions to find what feels best.

Myth: It's more tiring

Truth: Someone's body shape and weight says nothing about their flexibility, fitness or endurance. How tiring sex is also depends on the kind of sex you're having. When it comes to hard and fast fucking, everyone will need a break at some point.

When it comes to sex itself, there are a few things to remember: get into a comfy position, try something else if it's not working or doesn't feel great, use toys and lube, try incorporating props like cushions or sex wedges to get your body into the best position, bring touch to your whole body to awaken sensation, pause if you're tired, drink water if it's a long sesh, use language that is affirming and safe, and follow pleasure. Fat, thick and curvy bodies are sexy and deserving of great sex and pleasure.

SEXY, KINKY FAT

Sexy Kinky Fat is one of the most memorable workshops I've attended. It was run by Sam Jacob and Gina Machado and covered fat activism, sex education and pleasure. At the end, we were all invited to find fat on our bodies and explore it with sensation and touch. We brought pleasure to an area we've been taught to loathe and ignore. It was intense and vulnerable and felt really good. For years, I ignored my stomach during sex, but in this workshop, touching my waist was erotic.

I invite you to do the same. Find fat on your body and look at it, touch it, stimulate it. Tickle, caress and bring awareness to it. Don't ignore it – find ways to enjoy it.

The workshop ended with food play, also known as sploshing. We were invited to experience food that is deemed 'naughty' or bad, like cakes, cream and pasta. I went for the creamy, jammy, spongy cake and my friend offered her stomach. I placed the cake on her stomach, slowly sat on it and watched it ooze across her skin as I gyrated the cream cake all over her. It was silly and joyous, and my friend said it was liberating and transformational watching me experience pleasure from her stomach – a part of her body that for so much of her life she had been taught to ignore or feel ashamed of. In that moment, pleasure was a tool for radical resistance against fatphobia; it was a tool for our activism and a way to reclaim years of oppressive and restrictive thinking and eating.

Look, I know abolishing fatphobia is not as simple as sitting on a cake, but learning edges can (and should) have elements of play.

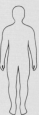

Body checking

How many times a day do you look at your body to evaluate and critique it? It's called body checking and it's a common practice for people who don't feel comfortable in their body. Our brains are hardwired to confirm what we expect to see, rather than observing what is present, so if we go to the mirror to check how bloated we are, we will fixate on that rather than seeing our body as a whole.

Body checking can have a knock-on effect for our sexual experiences, because we become hyper-aware of how our bodies look instead of how they feel. Sex becomes a performance, not an experience.

Next time you notice yourself doing a body check, bring your awareness to how you were feeling before, during and after the body check. Try reflecting on the following questions:

Did your emotional experience change at all?

How did your behaviour change?

If this habit is consuming or affecting you on a regular basis, it is important to seek support. For anyone who is wanting to build body acceptance and confidence, addressing body checking is a really important step.

As an experiment, I invite my clients to keep a tally of how often and for how long they check their bodies. We then add this tally up to see how much time is spent each day. It's often far longer than they'd like.

Draw up a table that looks like this. Try filling it out with your own body-checking habits that you want to adjust. I've filled it in as an example.

Body-checking behaviour	How often	Goal
Looking at stomach Assessing skin Asking people how I look Fixing hair Pinching skin	Twenty times a day	Twice a day – when I'm getting ready in the morning and before a meeting

You can start to work towards your goal gradually by setting incremental milestones or doing it all at once immediately.

Then let's realign our values. Yes, we can't ignore that appearance is important to many, especially if you value looking and feeling good. But what else do you value? Being kind, funny, intelligent, driven, compassionate, a great communicator, an amazing kisser? There is so much more to you than just your body; don't let the patriarchy distract you or preoccupy your mind, making you believe your worth is only derived by the way you look. When we start to understand our emotions and the behaviours that result from them, we have more choice over how we engage with our bodies.

IMPORTANT STUFF

✳ A big part of building confidence is finding your learning edge. You'll need to start doing the things that feel clunky or slightly uncomfortable. It's challenging at times, so make sure you're reflecting on all the good, useful work you're doing and give yourself a pat on the back ffs. And if you can't celebrate yourself, let me do it for you. It's tough stuff, but it's worth it.

✳ Building sexual confidence is a process – there is no quick fix – but this process can be fun, joyous, sexy and liberating.

✳ The best sexual partners are curious, playful and attuned. Sexual confidence comes with acknowledging that you don't need to be an expert in someone's body to be really fucking good at sex.

✳ Developing your sexual confidence may feel clunky and challenging at times, but the process can also be filled with pleasure, freedom and full-body-sponge-cake orgasms.

PLEASURE ZONES AND AROUSAL

Here is all the pleasure anatomy you need for great sex, solo and together: from the G-spot (which isn't actually a spot, but we'll get to that) to the clitoris, to the prostate and the A-spot. You'll learn how to start exploring your genitals and why you should spend time looking at them. We'll also geek out on the science of arousal: why it happens and what to do if you're not feeling aroused in the way you want to be.

In this book, you'll hear me talk about erogenous zones a lot. An erogenous zone is a part of the body that is sensitive to sexual stimulation. When we talk about erogenous zones, we're essentially talking about the zones of the body that turn you on.

Erogenous Zones

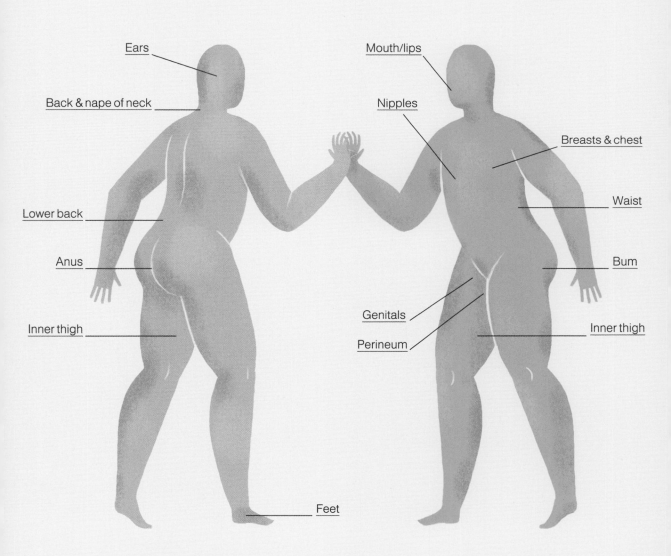

Ears

Back & nape of neck

Lower back

Anus

Inner thigh

Feet

Mouth/lips

Nipples

Breasts & chest

Waist

Bum

Genitals

Perineum

Inner thigh

Sure, there are some go-to areas that a lot of people find sexually stimulating, but you'll probably find that you have a few specific, perhaps surprising, places that turn you on when they're touched or stimulated. Some examples of the more recognised erogenous zones are nipples, chest, mouth, back, legs and inner thighs, ears, lips, bum, anus, genitals, neck and stomach. It may sound like I've listed pretty much every area in the body, and I guess I have. But there are also some surprising areas, such as nostrils, navel, hands and feet. In the right context and with the desired stimulation, the whole body has the capacity to be an erogenous zone.

Context can be a lot more important than you think. You may understand this if you've ever been in the same room as someone you're attracted to, and have experienced arousal without them even touching you. Just the heat of their body, knowing they're close, or them touching a typically non-sexual part of your body, such as brushing your arm, can be all it takes. Later in this chapter, we'll look at the science behind this, and how to integrate your whole body into sexual experiences. But for now, we're going to focus on the genitals.

Awareness of anatomy is the foundational tool for pleasurable sex. We're all told that genitals are the hub of pleasure and a key player in sex, but most of us have never been taught what makes the genitals erogenous zones.

So let's get into it. Here's a breakdown of the different pleasure zones in the genitals. This doesn't go into reproductive function – the focus here is on pleasure and sensation.

VULVA – EXTERNAL

The word 'vulva' refers to the external part of the genitals: so, the clitoris, labia and vaginal opening are all part of the vulva. For decades, medical textbooks were full of diagrams of the penis but contained no information about the clitoris. Pleasure for people with vulvas was largely ignored by science until the first in-depth study of the clitoris was led by Australian urologist Professor Helen O'Connell and published in 1998.

Mons pubis

An area of soft tissue that covers the pubic bone. It may or may not be covered in pubic hair.

The Vulva

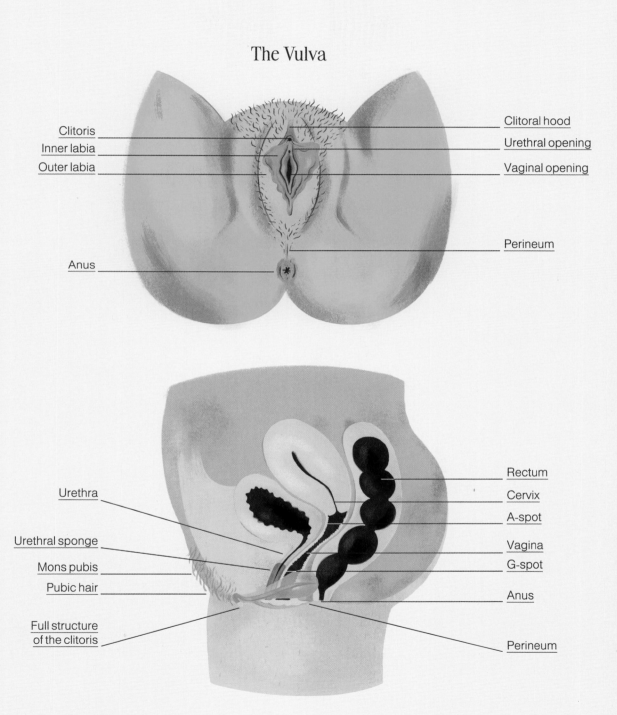

Clitoris

Inner labia

Outer labia

Anus

Clitoral hood

Urethral opening

Vaginal opening

Perineum

Urethra

Urethral sponge

Mons pubis

Pubic hair

Full structure
of the clitoris

Rectum

Cervix

A-spot

Vagina

G-spot

Anus

Perineum

Outer and inner labia

The outer labia are closest to the inner thighs; these are the 'lips', where pubic hair can grow. There is also an inner pair of labia, which are made up of more delicate tissues. Labia can be many colours, shapes and sizes, and they are often not symmetrical. Some people have larger outer labia, while others' inner labia may extend out. There are no 'normal' labia, just like there is no 'normal' nose.

Clitoral glans

Follow the line of the inner labia upwards, to a bean-like organ – this is the glans, or the head of the clitoris. It may seem small, but this tiny organ is home to most of the nerve endings in the genitals. The clitoris is typically protected by a clitoral hood, which is a thin membrane of skin. Gently pull the hood back to see or stimulate the clitoris. This is only the tip of the iceberg – the clitoris has legs and bulbs that extend into the body. More on this in the 'Internal' section.

Urethral opening

The urethral opening sits between the clitoris and the vaginal opening. This is the hole you wee from. The urethral opening is tiny, like a pinprick; not all people will be able to see it. This opening has a lot of sensitive tissue on either side of it. This is an erogenous zone, and is often referred to as the U-spot. With desired stimulation, it can feel incredibly pleasurable.

Perineum

Also referred to as 'the gooch', the perineum is the area between the vaginal opening and the anus. It has an internal network of erectile tissue, meaning any anal penetration or massage stimulates the clitoral network from new, highly sensitive angles.

Anus

The anus is surrounded by sensitive nerve endings and when stimulated it can feel pleasurable, deeply relaxing and even orgasmic. The pudendal nerve runs through the perineum – the area between the anus and the genitals – and branches out into other parts of the body, such as the genitals, pelvic floor muscles and anus. This complex nerve network makes the perineum sensitive to stimulation – so sometimes when you're experiencing anal stimulation, you feel it in your genitals as well.

INTERNAL EROGENOUS ZONES

Vagina

The vaginal opening is between the urethral opening and the perineum. The vagina is the muscular canal that connects the uterus to the vulva. In exploration, some may choose to insert fingers or a sex toy into the vagina. At the end of the vagina is the cervix, which opens up into the uterus, fallopian tubes and ovaries. Everyone's vagina is different in length.

Skene's glands

The Skene's glands are secretory glands located near the urethra. Research is yet to clarify what ejaculating, squirting and gushing actually are, but some studies suggest that the fluid produced before, during or after orgasm may be from the Skene's glands. Everyone with a vulva has the mechanics to squirt, but this doesn't mean that everyone will, or wants to. It's like orgasm: sometimes it happens, sometimes it doesn't. This involuntary emission of fluid is part of a broad spectrum of sexual responses and experiences.

The Clitoris

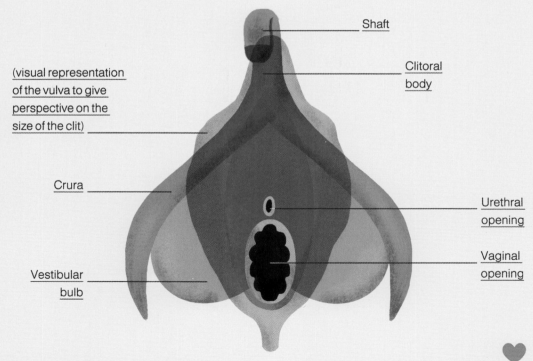

Shaft

Clitoral body

(visual representation of the vulva to give perspective on the size of the clit)

Crura

Vestibular bulb

Urethral opening

Vaginal opening

Clitoris

The clitoris is much larger than we can see – the majority of it is not usually visible. There are many things we're still discovering about this organ, but one thing we know for sure is its function: pleasure. The clitoris is made up of glans, a shaft and a body. The clitoral body extends upwards into the pelvis and attaches via ligaments to the pubic bone. From the clitoral body (located in front of the urethra), the clitoris forms the paired crura, aka the 'legs' of the clitoris and vestibular bulbs. The bulbs and crura contain erectile tissue that swells with blood during arousal. This swelling on either side of the vaginal canal can increase lubrication in the vagina, intensifying pleasure and sensation. The engorgement of clitoral tissue can also apply pressure on the G-spot.

G-spot

The G-spot isn't actually a spot, it's a part of the clitoral network. This means when you're stimulating the G-spot, you're also stimulating part of the clitoris from a new angle. It's more of an area or a zone than a magical spot and it's located on the front wall of the vagina. You can feel this area by inserting a finger into the vagina with the palm facing up, using a 'come hither' motion. When not aroused, it kind of feels like the roof of the mouth: rough and ridgey. When aroused, it can feel like the inside of a cheek: dense, spongy and soft. During arousal, the urethral sponge (which Sheri Winston coined the 'groove tube', because it's a tube of erectile tissue that wraps around the urethra), engorges and becomes erect. It protrudes from the vaginal wall, which makes the G-spot or zone feel more pleasurable and sensitive to touch, and for some, this stimulation can make them orgasm, but most people will need some type of external clit stimulation at the same time.

A-spot

If you explore deeper inside the vagina, you may be able to stimulate the A-spot, which is near the cervix. It's called the A-spot because it's on the anterior fornix, which means the front side of the body. Some people can reach it with their fingers, others may choose to use a toy.

Cervix

The cervix is a small passageway connecting the vagina to the lowest part of the uterus. The cervix looks like puckered lips, with a hole in the middle. The cervix moves, and changes in texture and position throughout the menstrual cycle. Not all people can reach their cervix with their fingers. This may be due to the length of their fingers, the length of the vaginal canal or the position they're in. During ovulation, the cervix may be higher and harder to reach. If you can reach it, don't be alarmed if you feel your cervix move. It is like a tongue, it can move around freely, but rest assured, it won't fall out. If you can't reach it, a toy may help you access it. You can experience deep pleasure with the desired stimulation of the cervix.

PENIS

People often assume the penis is simpler than the vulva because it is outside of the body. And while, sure, many people enjoy stroking the shaft, there's a lot more to penis pleasure than just a few rubs. Let's take a look.

Shaft

The shaft is also referred to as the 'body' of the penis. It's the area between the body and the head or glans of the penis. The shaft has three cylinders of erectile tissue – two are corpora cavernosa, and the other is corpus spongiosum. When aroused, the shaft engorges, becomes erect and often gets bigger, harder and longer in size.

Glans

The glans is basically the 'head' of the penis, and it is one of the most sensitive, and often pleasurable, areas of the penis. Some people enjoy direct stimulation of the glans, while others may find it too intense to have it directly massaged, touched, licked or sucked. The opening of the urethra sits at the tip of the glans and is sometimes referred to as the U-spot. It is a highly sensitive and pleasurable area.

Frenulum

Commonly and colloquially referred to as the 'banjo string', the frenulum is a fold or tissue, which kinda looks like a string, on the underside of the penis. The purpose of it is to allow the foreskin to be pulled back. It can also feel extremely pleasurable to touch and stimulate – some people can even climax from frenulum stimulation alone.

The Penis

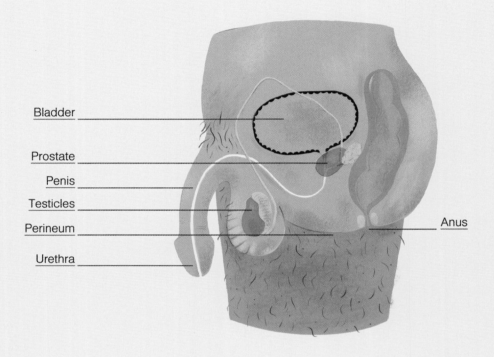

Bladder

Prostate

Penis

Testicles

Perineum

Urethra

Anus

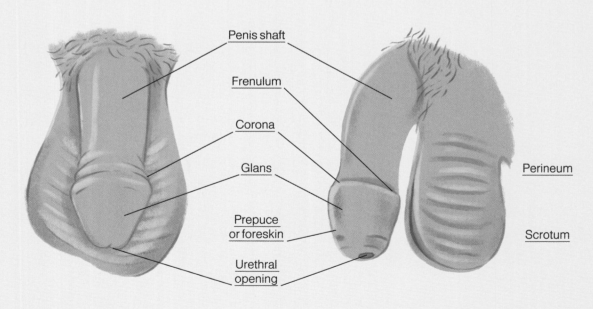

Penis shaft

Frenulum

Corona

Glans

Prepuce
or foreskin

Urethral
opening

Perineum

Scrotum

Scrotum

The scrotum is also referred to as the sac, because, as the name suggests, it's a sac of skin that holds the testicles and hangs in front of the body, between the legs. It's really sensitive, and many people enjoy it being, tickled, held and played with (gently at first) during sex.

Testicles

Also known as testes, balls, gonads, the testicles are two oval-shaped organs that produce and store sperm. They also produce hormones, the main one being testosterone. The testicles are very sensitive, and for this reason it can feel intensely pleasurable to receive touch and stimulation during sex.

Perineum

Also referred to as 'the gooch', this is the area between the scrotum and the anus. It contains an internal network of erectile tissue. Any anal stimulation, both internal and external, can feel incredibly pleasurable. Many people can experience a full-body, intense experience of pleasure that doesn't have to involve any penis stimulation and may not end in ejaculation.

Prostate

The prostate is a highly sensitive, walnut-sized gland often accessed through anal penetration. The function of the prostate is to secret prostate fluid, which is a component of semen, aka cum. For people with penises, this area can be a source of intense pleasure. Some people will orgasm from stimulating this area without ever ejaculating.

ARE MY GENITALS NORMAL?

At some point, most of us have asked, *Are my genitals are normal? Do they look, taste, smell or perform like everyone else's?* I often hear from people who feel insecure about their genitals. This is a result of a few factors, including the lack of diversity shown in porn, and airbrushing of genitals in ads, magazines and pop culture. Even Australian censorship guidelines state: 'Realistic depictions of sexualised nudity should not be high in impact. Realistic depictions may contain discreet genital detail but there should be no genital emphasis.'

Genital diversity: we're all different and that's normal

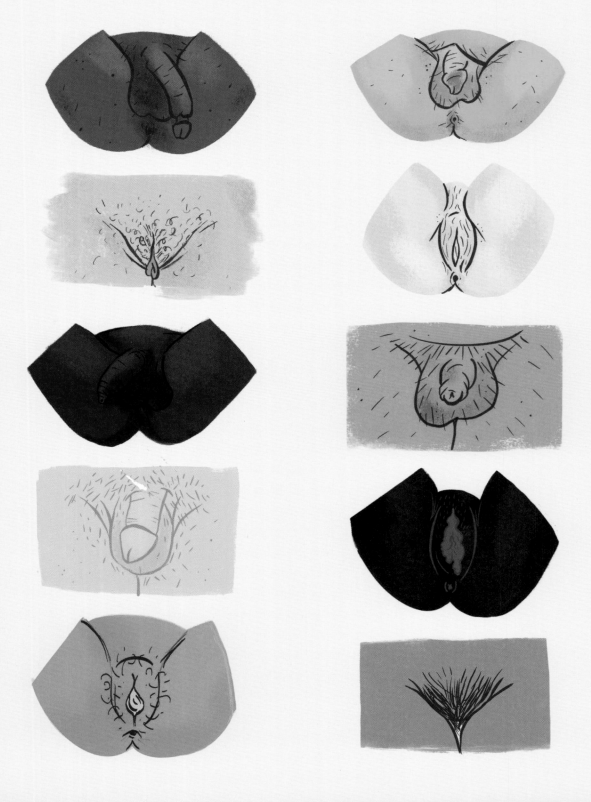

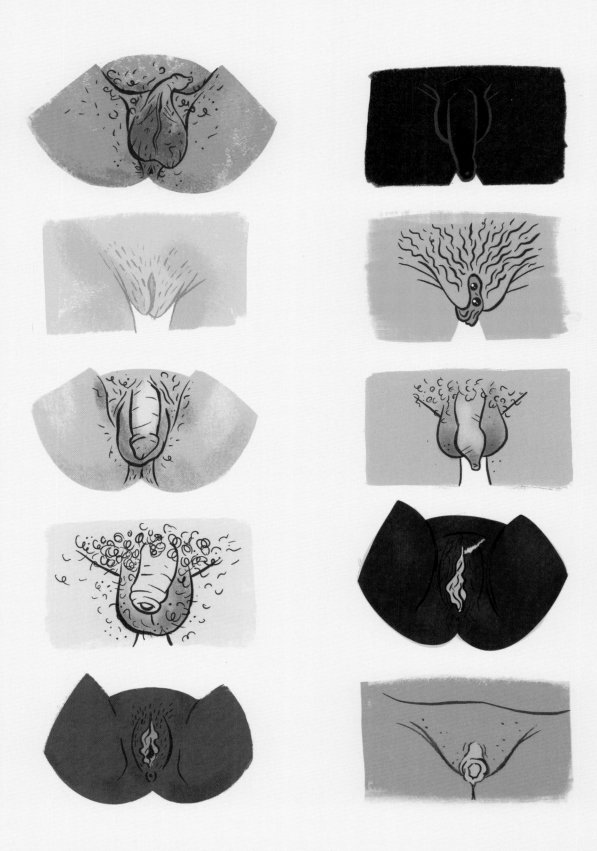

These guidelines mean there's limited awareness of diversity in genitals. Without access to inclusive, realistic images of genitals, many people think there is something wrong with them, which can lead to feelings of shame. Shame and sex are often relentless bed buddies. Feeling shame about your body is rarely useful. When we're ashamed of something – be it a fantasy, a desire or even a body part – we're typically reluctant to look at, touch or even acknowledge the source of our shame.

When we feel shame about our genitals, it's like having a blank space from the belly button down. This can have enormous impacts on our sexual experience. Some people may struggle to experience pleasure. It can also affect how present they can be during sex, and can have an ongoing emotional, physical and mental impact.

Internally, there are similarities between all genitals. Here you can see that the clitoris (left) and penis (right) are more similar than we've been led to believe.

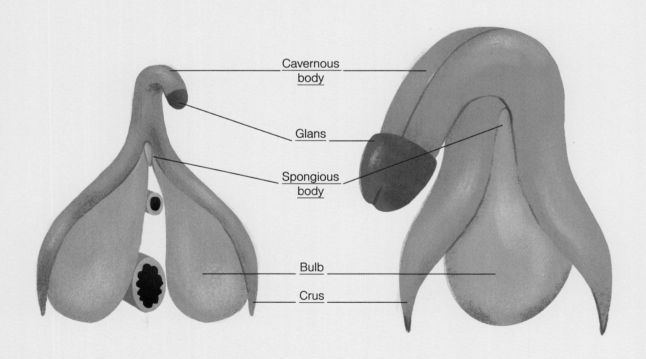

Cavernous body

Glans

Spongious body

Bulb

Crus

GENITAL FACTS

* There's no evidence to suggest vaginas 'get loose' after having lots of penetrative sex. This messaging is harmful and medically inaccurate. Vaginas don't get loose with each sexual partner, just like penises don't shrivel or shrink into flattened tissue with each sexual partner.

* Genitals smell like genitals, they are not meant to smell like flowers.

* All genitals are completely different, just like our faces.

* Genitals are rarely symmetrical – again, just like our faces.

* Sometimes our genitals don't perform the way we want them to – that's normal.

I once had a client who came to see me before she booked in for a cosmetic labiaplasty; our sessions were what she called her last chance to feel better about her vulva. She had grown up hearing teenage boys describe vulvas with graphic and horrible terms like a kebab or ham sandwich. This kind of language can have a lasting and devastating impact on many, affecting how comfortable they feel being naked, and their capacity to receive and feeling worthy of pleasure.

While we may think about our own genitals a lot and whether other people will like them, in reality very few of us are concerned about the appearance of our sexual partner's genitals. In fact, I've never had a client mention they're affected by their sexual partner's inner labia – and, believe me, people share some pretty vulnerable things. It's worth examining the messages we hear about 'normal' genitals. Ask yourself: *What has informed my idea of 'normal' genitals? How does it still affect me? In what ways is this unreasonable, unrealistic or unhelpful?*

Sexual shame can make us tap out of things we actually want. When we avoid situations or experiences because we're concerned about how our genitals look, we miss out on fun, meaningful, pleasurable moments. We reduce our bodies to something that must look perfect in order to experience pleasure. This then affects how we feel in our relationship with our own body and with others. We need to start disrupting this avoidance cycle. I know this can feel daunting, but it's often an important step.

The avoidance cycle

When we're anxious, we pay attention to a potential threat, then we become hyper-vigilant to possible signs of the threat. We feel like we can't or won't cope – and one way to reduce or ease this anxiety is to avoid it. Avoiding the threat leads to an instant decrease in anxiety in the short term but this can add to increased anxiety in the long term. This, my friends, is the avoidance cycle. And I regularly see this play out in my clients' relationships with their bodies.

When you feel anxious about, for example, your genitals, you may avoid looking at them or touching them because it feels too stressful. This helps you avoid the potential distress, so in the short term, you're not anxious (small win). But in the long term, you may become increasingly anxious about your genitals and continue to avoid them.

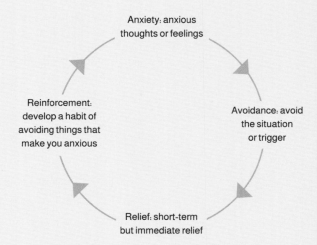

To disrupt this cycle, we need to gradually confront the feared situations. I recommend doing this with graded exposure so you can stay with your learning edge without pushing yourself too far. You might start by looking at your genitals while you have clothes on, then the next time without clothes on, then you might touch your genitals, then you might look at your genitals while touching them. This gradual approach can help you build confidence with your body and challenge the fear you have. By doing this in a structured and repeated way you can work to reduce anxiety. You may recognise it wasn't as bad as you thought it would be. And it may actually feel good.

It's important to create a safe environment in which we can start to reverse that cycle of avoiding our body. To disrupt the cycle we need to approach the situation.

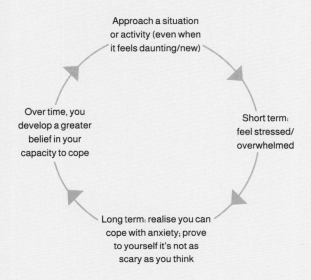

Approach a situation or activity (even when it feels daunting/new)

Short term: feel stressed/ overwhelmed

Long term: realise you can cope with anxiety; prove to yourself it's not as scary as you think

Over time, you develop a greater belief in your capacity to cope

This can feel really clunky and awkward at first – it always does when we're at our learning edge. Where to start will be different for everyone. Say, for example, someone feels uncomfortable receiving pleasure from a partner. In this case, they may start with masturbation, so they can practice receiving pleasure from themself.

Doing the daunting thing exposes us to a corrective experience. We can break the act down, and it doesn't have to be as scary as we're anticipating. From here, we keep moving the learning edge and adding in new challenges – for example, trying this practice in front of a mirror, or inviting a partner into the experience and guiding their hands.

AROUSAL

Now that you know where to stimulate, let's look at why we get turned on – or not – and how to build arousal to make sex feel even better.

Sexual arousal refers to the physiological changes that you experience as a result of stimulation. These changes could include an erect penis or clitoris, engorged or lubricated genitals, swollen nipples and breasts, an increased heart rate, flushed cheeks and even your pain threshold doubling. Signs of arousal can appear more quickly for people with penises than for those with vulvas. A penis can get erect in a few seconds, but a clitoris and vulva can take 20 to 40 minutes to be fully physiologically aroused. I can hear you yelling, FORTY MINUTES? I DON'T HAVE TIME FOR THAT! Don't worry, you can still have great sex and even climax in under 20 minutes , especially if you're using your favourite vibrator. I'm just referring to full genital arousal.

People with vulvas aren't complicated nor do they take too long to build arousal. Rather than trying to fix them and make them climax quicker, let's 'fix' the way we understand arousal and the way we engage in foreplay. To do this, it's useful to understand what's going on in the brain and body.

Dual-control model

Our sexual response is made up of two systems: the sexual excitation system (SES) and the sexual inhibition system (SIS).

The sexual excitation system is the **accelerator** for your sexual response. It scans your environment for everything you see, hear and feel, and sends signals from the brain telling the genitals to accelerate, or turn on. This can also operate beyond your consciousness, which explains those times when you find yourself thinking, *I have no idea why I'm turned on right now.*

Signals that can trigger the SES might include:

* the smell of someone's perfume or aftershave
* a knowing look or flirty smile
* a touch on your lower back
* context, such as being in an idyllic setting
* seeing someone attractive
* a really long, sensual back massage
* a hot, passionate kiss.

The sexual inhibition system is the **brake**. Research has found that there are two brakes within the SIS:

1. One brake scans your environment to stop you from getting aroused in contexts that may be inappropriate. This might include times when you know someone may hear you, when you're stressed about work, at a family event or in the middle of a task that needs to be done. Basically, it's your brain saying, 'Hey mate, not a good time right now.'

2. The other brake is what sex educator and researcher Emily Nagoski refers to as a 'handbrake'. It's a low-level 'no thank you', often driven by a fear of performance anxiety, such as not being able to climax, cumming too quickly or not being hard enough. This is really common. For example, if someone is worried that they won't get hard, their anxiety will then affect their erection.

This model can help us understand sexual function and dysfunction by identifying whether there's an imbalance between the brakes and accelerators. If you're currently struggling with arousal or sexual response, is it because you're riding the brakes or not getting enough acceleration? Getting aroused is a very individual thing. Try mapping out on a piece of paper what turns you on (accelerators) and what turns you off (brakes).

Feeling aroused is the process of turning on the 'ons' and turning off the 'offs'. This is a foundational skill that many of us are not aware of, and very few of us have been taught how to do. We just sit and wait for it to appear. But often to feel motivated for sex we need to engage with specific accelerators and manage or remove the brakes. We'll build on this when we get to Chapter 11.

WHAT IF I DON'T FEEL AROUSED WHEN I WANT TO?

There's this assumption that when you're attracted to someone or in love with them, you should be able to get erect, wet and turned on at the drop of a hat. It can be confusing when you want sex but you are not getting aroused. And on the flip side, you may have also experienced being physiologically aroused but not wanting or desiring sex. This is what we call arousal non-concordance – when our bodies respond in unexpected ways. Nagoski states, 'Arousal non-concordance is the well-established phenomenon of a lack of overlap between how much blood is flowing to a person's genitals and how "turned on they feel".' This is why you can't always turn to your genitals to determine whether you want sex. The only thing that can determine whether you want to have sex is you. Not your erection, vaginal lubrication, hard nipples, or anything else. Only you.

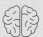

Examine and challenge

It's important to understand the cultural, social and political influences on the way we feel about our bodies, and to consider how we might draw on some of the following approaches to rewire a disgust response and build a safe relationship.

* Reflect on the messages you've received about bodies – where have these ideas come from?

* Learn about genital diversity and do your research.

* Examine and challenge the not-so-useful thoughts about your relationship with your genitals.

* Observe how you speak about your body. Focus on sensation, pleasure and function over aesthetics.

* Build awareness of your body through touch, masturbation and pleasure.

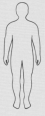

Look at your genitals – it's good for you

Looking at your genitals, or even just your body, can be confronting, I know. It's not uncommon to feel disconnected or ashamed. But the more you know about your genitals, the more awareness you will have. More awareness leads to more sensation, and more sensation leads to more pleasure. Examining your genitals can be a great learning tool, and not enough people do it. It can allow you to access more pleasure in your body, and it can also feel incredibly healing. A great way to do this is through mirror work. This is a way to heal, develop self-love, learn about your body and build a more dynamic relationship with it.

For this exercise all you need is a safe space, a hand-held mirror that you can put in front of (you may also like props to support your positioning), body-safe lube of choice, and at least ten minutes. Now, let's get started.

* Breathe. (Flick back to Chapter 2 if you need a reminder of how to use your breath to become present.)

* Look down at your genitals, then move your gaze to the mirror so that you can see more.

* Gaze at your genitals for however long you like.

You may stop the enquiry here, but if you're curious and want to explore more, try this.

* Locate the different parts of your genitals. Understand which parts of your genitals might feel sensitive, and think about how you would communicate this to a partner.

* Explore these organs or areas with a variety of touch, pressure or sensation.

* Integrate the experience with a few mindful moments, or by journalling about the process.

* Follow pleasure. See if you can find pleasurable ways of stimulating each part of your genitals. This is an exploration to build awareness – it doesn't have to feel orgasmic. You might like to stroke, caress, gently pinch, soothe, touch or rub your genitals. Do this for however long you like.

It's not for everyone, but some people like to use affirmations, or speak as they explore their genitals, offering gentle reminders to themselves that this is normal and safe. Allow yourself to feel whatever comes up. There is no right or wrong way to experience this practice. After you've done this on your own, you may choose to do this with a partner.

When your body doesn't respond the way you want

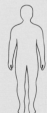

It can be frustrating and confusing when your body responds in unexpected ways, but there's a lot you can do.

* Slow it right down, pause or stop. By slowing down, you can come back to the sensation that is present. Hard and fast sex is great, but often you need to build arousal in your body first for it to feel really good. Also, let's normalise taking a break or stopping – this is normal, and helps us recalibrate. It doesn't need to be a smooth contemporary dance in the sheets.

* Tell your partner about what turns you on and off. If they don't know, they can't give it to you – and I promise you, people want to know how to pleasure you best. (If they're not interested, that's a larger conversation.) Tell them where, how and what you like – be descriptive to the point of it feeling uncomfortable. Even if you've been together a long time, these things can evolve, and you might need to communicate how they've changed.

✳ Actively create the context for arousal on a more regular basis. Think about your accelerators, what does your body need to build arousal? How many brakes are present and what can you do to manage or remove them?

✳ Create an arousal toolkit. This could include things like lube, toys and sensory items. Sometimes, as much as we like to think we've got it all, lube and toys are one way to make sex reliably great. Use lube. Every single time you masturbate or have sex.

✳ Ask questions. What would make this better? How do you like to touch yourself?

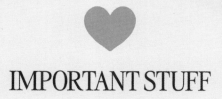

IMPORTANT STUFF

✳ Your genitals are normal.

✳ Learning about pleasure anatomy is a foundational tool for great solo and partnered sex. So take your time to locate and explore sensation.

✳ The more aroused you are, the better sex will feel, so it's important to take time to build arousal in your body.

✳ If your body isn't responding the way you think it should, or the way you want it to, there could be a reason for this – arousal non-concordance.

✳ Genitals look, smell and taste like genitals. They're not meant to be a rose or a raspberry-scented candle.

MASTURBATION

Whether you're a beginner or a seasoned professional, you can always learn more and experience more through masturbation. This chapter explains how to level up your masturbation, how to incorporate aids like sex toys, and how to create a pleasure map of your body.

For many of us, masturbation is one of our first sexual experiences. That might have been humping a pillow, a surprising encounter with a shower head or rubbing one out into a sock. Despite it being common, normal and even beneficial to our sex lives, we're never really taught how to masturbate well. So instead, we turn to porn, media or friends. Fortunately, this act that was once considered shameful is increasingly being celebrated as a vital part of human sexuality. However, there are some enduring misconceptions, which affect how people feel about it.

COMMON MISCONCEPTIONS

Myth: You'll ruin yourself for partnered sex

Truth: If anything, masturbation will make partnered sex better. It helps you learn about your body, what you like and how you want to be touched, and this can make it easier to communicate wants and needs with a sexual partner. There's also no scientific evidence to suggest people desire partnered sex less because they're too used to pleasuring themselves.

Myth: You'll become infertile

Truth: There's no evidence to suggest masturbation affects fertility. While it was once thought that wanking could lower sperm count, this is not true – the body continually produces sperm, so you won't run out. In fact, regularly masturbating can actually be a useful tool as it can help you feel less stressed, more relaxed and more in touch with your body, which is actually useful for those trying to conceive.

Myth: You'll get acne, your palms will be hairy, you'll go blind

Truth: There's ZERO evidence – none, zip, zilch – that suggests masturbation will cause blindness, hairy palms or acne. Think about how many people masturbate worldwide on a daily basis. Now, how many hairy palms did you last see on your way into work?

These myths are rooted in a culture of sexual shame, which warns that sex is meant to be between a man and a woman who love each other very much and must not be for – god forbid! – pleasure. But I'm here to tell you, there are so! many! benefits! to masturbating. It is a vital tool for learning about your body, it's a great source of stress relief, it releases feelgood neurochemicals, it can support us in feeling more connected to our bodies, it can bring sex front of mind and in turn help us desire sex more, it can be used as a tool to help overcome sexual dysfunction like pre-orgasmia, erectile dysfunction and premature ejaculation, and that's just the beginning. There are endless benefits.

It's also a very valid experience of sex in itself – after all, solo sex is sex! The better you know your body, the easier it is for you to communicate your wants, needs, and desires. Exploratory masturbation supports the process of neuroplasticity, the networks in our brain that change when we engage in new behaviours.

This alone expands our capacity to feel. Everyone can benefit from a solid masturbation practice.

Another misconception is that masturbation is something you only do by yourself. In Chapter 12, we'll explore mutual masturbation and how it can be used to achieve more pleasure and longevity in partnered sex. But first, let's focus on you.

BREATH AND MASTURBATION

Breath is your erotic pump – you can use your breath to build/pump up your arousal, as well as decrease or release it – and has many benefits when it comes to sex. It can help you:

✳ build and regulate arousal

✳ feel more connected

✳ reduce stress and tension

✳ feel more sensation

✳ be more present

✳ reset the nervous system

✳ feel more connected to others.

So many people tense up, clench their body and hold their breath when they have sex, almost clawing their way to orgasm.

Breath is an essential tool, as it has an immediate physiological effect on your body. Try it for yourself. Take a deep breath now and lengthen your exhale. How do you feel? Breath is one of the quickest ways to physiologically change the way we're feeling. There are so many exercises you can do. Often, breathwork practices fall into two categories: up-regulating and down-regulating breath.

UP-REGULATING

This breathing technique will help you build arousal. Here are a few foundational practices to start with. If you feel light-headed, stop, sit down and lengthen your exhale.

✳ **Fast inhale:** Quickly suck your breath in through pouted or pursed lips. Start with no more than ten rounds, as this can make you feel light-headed.

✳ **Breath and movement:** Sync your breath with movement; try something like a hip thrust.

✳ **Breathe and engage your pelvic floor:** As you breathe, engage and release your pelvic floor muscles (these are the muscles you engage when you want to stop a wee mid-stream). Engage on an inhale and on an exhale, release.

✳ **Synchronise your breathing:** Before you have sex with someone else, it can feel connecting and arousing to sync your inhales and exhales.

DOWN-REGULATING

Down-regulating, as you may have guessed, is the opposite (kind of) to up-regulating. You can use down-regulated breathing to help you move away from arousal, so it is an essential tool for people trying to last longer during sex. If at any point it feels uncomfortable, stop, sit down and come back to your regular breath.

✳ **Box breath:** Breathe in for four seconds, hold for four seconds, exhale for four seconds, hold for four seconds. Imagine you're breathing to the four sides of a box.

✳ **Deep and long:** Breathe from your abdomen. Imagine your lower stomach is a balloon, using the contraction of your stomach muscle to inhale and exhale.

✳ **Lengthen the exhale:** Make your exhale last a few counts longer than your inhale.

✳ **Breathe with a sigh and sound:** Ever sighed and had it feel like a perfect release? Making sound can feel really down-regulating. On each exhale, make a sound. This could be a soft sigh or a moan. Explore what feels right.

I teach these two basic categories of breathing exercises to my clients. You won't learn or experience anything new from just reading those practices. Give them a try, at first in a non-sexual environment and then start implementing them into sex with yourself or others.

GREAT SOLO SEX AND SETTING THE CONTEXT

Often when we masturbate, we're so quick to just make it happen, orgasm and wipe off. And there's certainly a time and a place for that. But masturbation can also be so much more. It sounds simple, but often my clients will say that some of their best solo sex experiences have come after they've taken time to create a sexual context, just like they'd set a sexual context if they were having sex with someone else. Think about the practical things you need to set the mood. How can you create the context for a good time? A few themes I hear often: locking the door, having a sensual shower, keeping toys and tools close by, awakening sensation in your whole body with a full body massage using your favourite cream or oil, creating a sex playlist, drawing the blinds, taking your time.

MASTURBATION POSITIONS TO TRY

Over the years you may have found a go-to technique or position that feels good for you. This is a great foundation, but the more you learn and explore, the more you expand your pleasure potential. Here are some illustrations of a few popular techniques and positions. This is not an exhaustive list. Start with these – some may feel great, others may not. There's a full breakdown of touch techniques in Chapter 12 that can be applied to solo or partnered sex.

AWARENESS AND MOVEMENT

Masturbation doesn't have to only be about getting off. It's actually a pretty powerful tool that can help to increase your own pleasure and the length of time you last before climax.

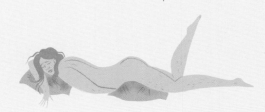

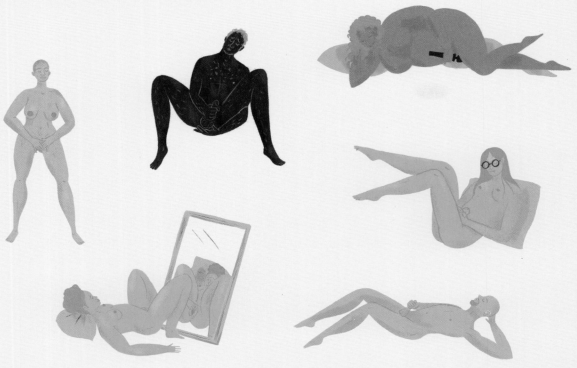

To increase pleasure during masturbation, try bringing attention to specific parts of your body. By heightening awareness, you can heighten pleasure.

Get your whole body into it. When most people masturbate, they are often tense and have very little movement in their bodies. A tension orgasm can feel good, but actually bringing movement and your whole body into it can enhance sensation. Try incorporating these movements:

✳ hip tilts: rocking your hips back and forth

✳ teasing: taking time to build arousal before going straight to the genitals

✳ edging: moving towards and away from orgasm

✳ pelvic floor exercises and movement: engaging and releasing your pelvic floor as you thrust your hips.

USING SEX TOYS

If you've never used toys before and you're not sure where to begin, I suggest flicking straight to Chapter 14 to get the full lowdown. Then come back here and keep reading.

Using a sex toy on your own doesn't have to be a quick experience focused solely on cumming. At least, not every time.
Start by using the toy to awaken sensation and build arousal in and around your whole body. Once you're ready to bring the toy to your genitals, make sure you use enough body-safe and toy-safe lube (the toy should specify which lubes are compatible).

Externally, you could try things like circles, up and down, or side to side. And if you're using a dildo or a prostate massager internally, you could try replicating the 'come here' motion, using the toy for penetration by moving it in and out. Try barrel rolling, pushing, or holding it with just the right amount of pressure in a zone that feels best for you. Try using vibration across erogenous zones. If you have a penis, try it on your frenulum, perineum or anus (externally); and if you have a vulva, try using vibration on the perineum, outer labia, vaginal opening, urethral opening. I'd also recommend bringing in movement practices. Sure, you could just turn it on, put it in place and get going, but you can intensify the sensation by bringing your whole body into the experience.

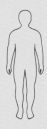

Mapping your body

People are often curious about new ways they can masturbate, or ways to increase pleasure and sensation. The very first step is learning about your body, and the best way to do that is to start exploring. This exploration can feel daunting at first – where to begin?

One starting point is with body mapping, a practice of mapping out sensation in your body through touch. Basically, you're viewing your body as a map and locating sensation. This is a useful practice for anyone who's feeling numb, disconnected or wanting to expand pleasure potential.

When you practise mapping often and with purpose, your overall awareness of your body will improve, allowing you to feel more in tune with pleasure. Here's how to do it:

⁂ Get comfortable and choose a body part you'd like to awaken, such as your hands, arm, stomach or genitals.

⁂ Set a timer for five minutes.

⁂ Bring touch to this body part and explore where it feels numb, nothing, pleasurable, good, etc.

⁂ Now slow it right down, then slow it down some more.

⁂ As you touch, breathe. Notice how you feel and what kind of touch you want to receive.

⁂ Follow any sensation that feels nice. Explore different types of pressure, movement and speed.

⁂ When the timer goes, stop touching and observe what you're feeling.

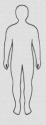

Seven days of masturbation

You may do these seven days in a row or once a month: do whatever feels best for you. These practices aren't about 'reaching' orgasm; they're about following pleasure.

✳ **Day one:** Mindful masturbation practice. You may want to start with a guided meditation or simply bring awareness to your breath, movement, sound and touch as you masturbate.

✳ **Day two:** Map your genitals externally to discover sensation (with or without a mirror).

✳ **Day three:** Map genitals or anus internally to discover pleasure and sensation.

✳ **Day four:** Map genitals or anus internally and externally for blended stimulation.

✳ **Day five:** Explore movement like hip tilts, grinding, body rolls or standing while you masturbate.

✳ **Day six:** Experiment with sensation and other tools, like toys or sensory items.

✳ **Day seven:** Freestyle! Follow what feels good for you.

Five ways to increase pleasure and longevity

1. Breath: up-regulating (fast) or down-regulating (slow) breaths.

2. Movement: hip thrusts when standing or lying down, sensual movement and/or dance.

3. Sounds: moans, sighs, audible exhales.

4. Touch: full body touch, exploring different pressures or stimulation.

5. Awareness: bring attention to specific parts of your body.

IMPORTANT STUFF

✳ Masturbation is a foundational tool for learning about pleasure in your own body and improving your sexual experience with others.

✳ There is nothing wrong or shameful about masturbation, and it won't ruin your sex life with others – if anything, it'll make it better.

✳ You can always learn new types of touch and explore new sensations by trying different techniques, positions and sensations. Moving beyond masturbation habits can help expand your pleasure potential.

✳ Breath doesn't often come to mind as a masturbation technique, but it can be an effective tool for feeling more, and for regulating your pleasure.

ORGASM

How can I make myself cum? Why do I cum so quickly? Am I doing it like everyone else? We have a social and cultural fascination with the big O. It makes sense – after all, orgasming feels really good – but chasing a ten-second crescendo can dampen your overall sexual experiences. In this section we'll cover the foundations of orgasm and address the most common climax concerns.

When I ask clients what an orgasm feels like, no two answers will be the same. An intense wave of pleasure, a disappointing release, like having an itch scratched, a full-body-leg-trembling explosion, too intense, scary, like losing all control, the best feeling in the world. We all feel orgasms differently, and they can also feel different each time. In fact, there isn't a single definition of what an orgasm actually is. That's because there's a lot to consider.

Orgasms are physiological, psychological, emotional and sexual. They're a peak moment in pleasure. Orgasms happen in the brain, but they're experienced through stimulation in certain parts of the body. People can experience orgasms in many ways – and they're not always sexual. People may experience orgasm through stimulating erogenous zones, but it's also really common to have a sleeping orgasm. Some may also climax through breathwork, although this is probably less common, and let's not forget the surprising phenomenon of an exercise-induced orgasm. (No, that doesn't mean you want to have sex with the treadmill.) They're not always going to be an eye-rolling, leg-trembling, divine-intervention style experience. In fact, sometimes it can just feel like a release, or a very gentle throb.

Orgasms are a common reason for having sex. People love them. They feel great. But while they can be incredibly pleasurable and exciting, they are also the very reason someone may book a session with a sex therapist. We're orgasm obsessed, and often not in the most useful way – orgasm has become something we need to achieve in order to know sex was good, or that we were good. The pressure to achieve this goal can be counterintuitive, as it takes us out of the moment entirely.

Understanding how they work, the different ways you can experience them and the phases of orgasm is often the first step to feeling more pleasure – and, ultimately, cumming.

THE PHASES OF ORGASM

Over the years, sex researchers have developed models to explain orgasm. Masters and Johnson's model from 1966 broke orgasm into four phases. Then in 1979, Kaplan's model included desire. You can see both models on the next page.

While these were revolutionary at the time, we now know that orgasm is a very individual thing. However, many of my clients still think this is how they should respond. They desire their partner, they want to have sex, so why are they not experiencing the sexual arousal and orgasm they so desperately want? The journey to orgasm is rarely linear or predictable, as it can be influenced by many factors. In fact, the work of Emily Nagoski has proved that arousal and desire are not the same thing. You can be physiologically aroused without wanting or desiring sex.

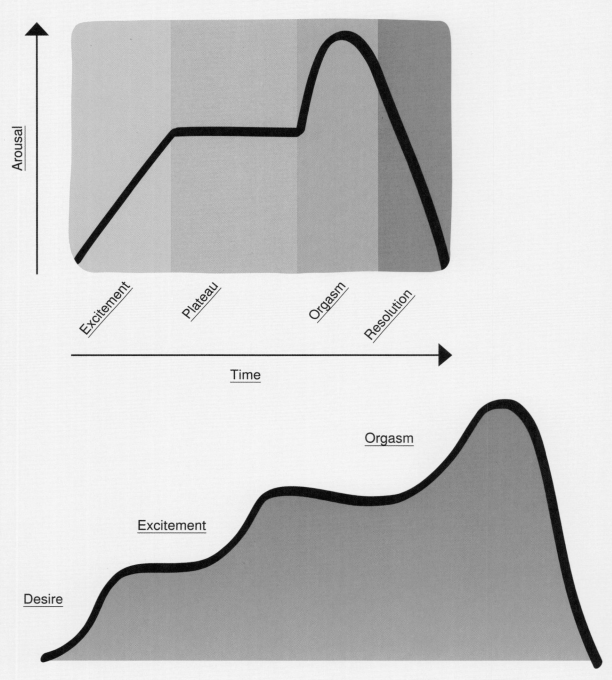

Masters and Johnson's Phases
of the Sexual Response Cycle, 1966

Arousal

Excitement

Plateau

Orgasm

Resolution

Time

Orgasm

Excitement

Desire

Kaplan's Triphasic Model
of Sexual Response, 1979

On the other hand, you may also want and desire sex without physically showing signs of arousal.

Sometimes our journey to orgasm can feel like this:

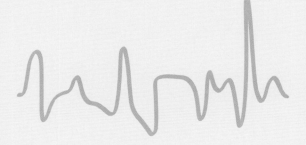

The next time you masturbate or have sex, take a moment afterwards to map out your own arousal graph. What did it look like for you?

PRE-ORGASMIA

Many people are familiar with the feeling of desperately wanting to orgasm but not quite getting there, or wanting to last longer but not being able to make it. Like many things with sex, it's an incredibly individual and normal thing to experience.

Anorgasmia refers to the inability to orgasm despite sexual stimulation. I don't use this term, because it essentially means you can't or won't orgasm. People tend to google the term and become fixated on the percentage of people who will never climax. Instead, I like the term 'pre-orgasmia', because it reinforces the idea that, sure, you haven't had an orgasm *yet*, but there's SO much you can do to explore pleasure in your body – maybe you just haven't found the right tools yet.

First up, I want to get clear on what some mean by 'can't cum'. I can't even tell you how many people claim they've never climaxed, when they actually climax with ease during masturbation and only struggle with it when there's penetration. Statistically, this is incredibly common; the majority of people with vulvas will only ever climax from external stimulation, and many aren't getting anywhere near enough.

When I'm working with clients, I like to approach this issue from a few angles: education, coaching, counselling and creating an action plan. Basic sex ed isn't always needed, but it's a good place to start. I like to teach people about anatomy, pleasure and orgasms as a base point. From there, we'll work on a coaching element. This involves skill-based practices like breath, movement, sound, touch and placement of awareness. I also go over how to masturbate in a way that invites sensation into the body.

Counselling and therapy can help you make sure you know why you're feeling things and how you're feeling them. In a session, we look into what's getting in the way of your pleasure. It could be stress, anxiety, shame or low sexual confidence. When we have figured this out, it's a lot easier to work on it.

Finally, we co-create an action plan. Yours might be 30 Days of Masturbation and its intention is to rewire neural pathways and allow for new experiences. You're not going to be able to magically climax without learning about your body and actually exploring pleasure.

Letting go and releasing into pleasure is a challenge for many. For some, pleasure may feel too intense. You might even feel like you're about to wee. If it ever feels too much, try to slow down, ease the pressure or even just pause for a moment, rather than backing off entirely, as this feeling is often a sign that you're about to 'get there'.

WHY IS MY BODY NOT RESPONDING THE WAY I THINK IT SHOULD?

The word 'should' comes up a lot in my sessions with clients. So often we have high standards for our bodies and what we think they should be doing. *This should feel good. This should make me cum.* Remember: everybody is different, every brain is different, and the way we respond to sexual stimulation is different too.

Awakening sensation in your body is doable, and an important part of feeling more pleasure. It's all about bringing awareness to a part of your body and stimulating it. Most of us have never been taught how to access or heighten pleasure. I like to work with a few practical somatic tools to improve the awareness of sensation: breath, movement, sound and touch. The practice I teach was developed by Dr Betty Martin. She calls it 'awakening sensation in the hands'. It's a powerful way to tap into an almost meditative state, to bring awareness to your body, and to learn about following pleasure and sensation in a way that isn't goal driven.

Give this a go – you're here to do things differently, after all. It'll only take five minutes.

✳ Close your eyes and focus your attention and awareness on your hands. Think about which hand will be 'giving' touch and which hand will be 'receiving' touch.

✳ Set a timer for five minutes, then try to awaken the sensation and feeling in the hand that is the receiver. Touch your palm, touch your fingers, trace around the space between them. You can touch, tickle, knead or slap every inch of your hand – just make sure to notice and explore how it feels.

✳ Once the timer goes off, stop touching your hand and spend a moment focusing on how both hands feel. What's different about them? What are you noticing? What are you feeling?

This practice is so simple, but people are often surprised by how much it brings awareness to sensations in their body. Some even feel aroused and turned on. I often ask my clients to practise this every day for a month. This supports people in recognising the role awareness brings to sensation. The hand has lots of rich nerve endings, but your genitals are even more sensitive – so why do we feel numb and disconnected from our genitals, but our hands can feel so much?

This practice also teaches us how to follow pleasure. And then we take this process and apply it to another erogenous zone – perhaps your neck, inner thighs or genitals. If you're keen to continue awakening sensation in your body, set your timer for ten minutes and choose an erogenous zone you're curious about. Bring the same curiosity and exploration to this body part as you did to your hands. Once your timer has gone off, take the time to focus on how you felt and what you noticed. We do this to connect your mind to the way your body physically feels things. This connection is incredibly important, and it is a learnable skill.

SEX VALUES

I will often work through a sex values pie chart (see examples on the next page) with my clients, particularly when high importance is placed on orgasm, which can add a lot of pressure to sex. In these cases, I'll show my clients the top circle. I'll say, 'This is all you're valuing about sex: orgasm. This one thing holds all the importance, but I have a sense that sex is so much more meaningful than just orgasm alone.' I'll then ask them why sex is important to them.

Write out your own sex values, and talk about them with others. Why do you have sex? Why is it important to you? Why did you buy this book to learn more?

There are so many things that drive us to sex. At some point, we all need to examine these things. What drives us to value it?

♥ 83

Sex Values

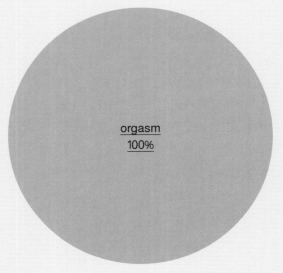

orgasm
100%

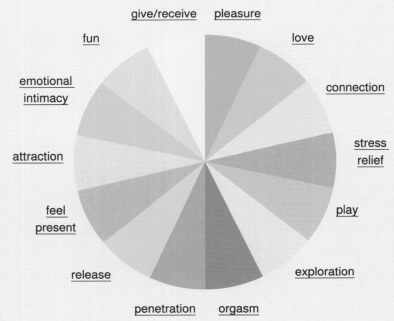

give/receive   pleasure
fun   love
emotional   connection
intimacy
                        stress
attraction   relief

feel   play
present
release   exploration

penetration orgasm

TAKE THE PRESSURE OFF

By the time someone comes to see me, they're often pretty stuck. So first up, let's take the pressure off. I invite many of my clients to take sex or orgasm off the table for an agreed period of time, as well as releasing any expectations and 'shoulds'. This may sound counterintuitive, but it can relieve a lot of pressure and allow you to do things that you want to do, rather than things you feel you should do.

They start to redefine sex. How can you invite intimate or pleasurable moments into your relationship beyond 'naked bodies penetrating each other'? A passionate kiss, a massage, jumping in the shower together – all of these things can be fulfilling sexual experiences. Start being intimate in ways that are exciting and fulfilling, and focus on the quality of the experience rather than the quantity or goal. Let's focus on the questions: what is possible/fun/sexy right now?

FAKING ORGASMS

Should you fake an orgasm? This is a pretty divisive question, and I don't think there's a blanket 'yes' or 'no' answer. Long story short, do whatever *you* want. It's your body, your experience, your pleasure, your way. It's more common for a person with a vulva to fake an orgasm than a person with a penis, maybe for the obvious reason that many people with penises ejaculate when they climax.

Faking orgasms can put someone else's satisfaction and ego over your own pleasure. People will put up with mediocre, boring or unfulfilling sex because they don't want their partner to feel bad or insecure, but this only repeats the idea that sex is a performance and that penetrative sex is king.

Over the years, I've noticed a few common reasons why people fake an O:

✳ They want sex to be over and done with.

✳ They haven't experienced orgasms and feel insecure or ashamed about it.

✳ They're concerned about taking too long.

✳ They don't want to make their partner insecure – they're prioritising their partner's satisfaction or self-esteem over their own pleasure.

✳ They're feeling pressure to perform.

✳ They're feeling uncomfortable receiving.

✳ They assume a good sexual experience needs to involve climax or a peak moment.

It is worth noting that some people find faking orgasm can help get them in the mood, turn themselves on, build arousal, allow for greater presence and increase fun/excitement. Some even climax at the sound of their own pleasure.

You're not a bad person for faking climax. You're not a bad feminist, or a bad sexual partner either. Sometimes we feel we don't have the tools or language to really communicate what we want. There's enough shame around sex – you will never catch me saying you're 'bad' or 'wrong' for faking an orgasm.

But if you're tempted to fake an O, it may be worth considering why you're inclined to do so – and what you can do instead to ensure you're having the best time possible, orgasm or not. If you want to get out of the habit and invite more pleasure into your life, try the following.

✳ **Communicate**. Learn ways to tell your sexual partner when the touch or stimulation is no longer hitting the spot or exciting for you. Be descriptive, clear and ongoing in your communication, and stop settling for 'okay'. Instead of willing sex to be over, use language like 'Can we try …' or 'I love it when you …' or 'I want you to …' or 'I'm not sure if this will feel good but can we explore …'

✳ **Take the orgasm off the pedestal.** Orgasms are an important part of sex, but they can also add a lot of pressure. You may find it useful to consider your sex values – i.e. the things that feel important during sex. Maybe orgasm is meaningful to you, but what else is valuable? Sensation, pleasure, playfulness, exploration, love, connection? By realigning our sex values, we take the pressure and focus off orgasm, leaving us free to enjoy the whole experience, rather than just a few seconds.

✳ **Focus on touching and being touched.** Sensate focus is a therapy technique developed by Masters and Johnson that invites people to come back to their senses and current desires/awareness and to move away from a goal-driven, penetration-focused idea of sex. You could start off touching everywhere except the genitals, then progress if it feels right. Ask yourself: *What would make this better? What feels good right now?* Come back to your body and the current sensations. Follow pleasure.

✳ **Try mutual masturbation.** This is a great way to demonstrate how you like to be touched – and it can also be really hot.

✳ **Use tools!** Toys, lube, sensory items … they all exist to make sex more pleasurable. Sex isn't just about two bodies penetrating each other. It can be anything you want.

✳ **Redefine the end of sex.** Sex doesn't always end in climax. Consider other ways of defining the conclusion of sex, such as setting a timer for a certain period of time, or just finishing when you're no longer into it.

ERECTILE DYSFUNCTION

If you or your partner suffers from ongoing erectile issues (i.e. it happens more than a few times) or all of a sudden you start struggling to get it up, it's important to see a GP, as erectile dysfunction can be an early indicator of cardiovascular disease.

Feeling stressed about how your body performs is so human, especially when it comes to sex. I find there's a lot of pressure on people who have penises to be rock hard and ready to go at all times, but our bodies don't always respond in the way we want them to. When someone is experiencing a sexual concern like this, it can have a huge impact on how they feel about themselves and sex in general and also how they relate to their partner.

Often people who are struggling with arousal experience so much shame and fear that their body won't respond in the way they want it to that they will stop having sex altogether. They stop kissing their partner, they stop telling them how attractive they are, they stop touching them, because they fear that if they engage in anything intimate or sexual then their partner may want to have sex with them, so they pull back from all intimacy. And then everyone misses out.

Living with a sexual concern such as premature ejaculation or erectile dysfunction can affect a person's whole sense of self. And it's not just something they think about when they're having sex. They think about it throughout the whole day. If they're dating, they may be nervous before they even go on a date, thinking about how they can avoid sex or trying to prepare themselves to perform for this new sexual partner.

These kinds of sexual concerns are incredibly common, and there is a lot that can be done to address them. Remember, there is no shame in seeking support.

If your body is responding in an unexpected way, go back to the tools we addressed in Chapter 2. These will support you in regulating arousal in a sexual context. Do these often outside of a sexual context, then in a sexual context try these things:

✳ **Stop, slow down or pause.** Instead of getting frustrated, or beating yourself up about it, come back to the pleasure and sensation that is present – this may mean going back to kissing.

✳ **Bring awareness back to pleasure.** Move your attention away from the goal of penetration and back to sensation that does feel good: the way your hand feels on your body – or if you're with someone else, the feeling of their skin or lips.

✳ **Breathe.** When we're stressed, it's very common to hold our breath, tense up and numb ourselves out. This can be as simple as lengthening your exhale for the count of four.

✳ **Use cock rings.** The function of a cock ring is to make your penis more erect. A vibrating cock ring can also feel pleasurable for the person you're penetrating.

✳ **Have sex that doesn't rely on penetration.** There is SO much you can explore; the more creative you are the better sex feels for everyone involved. Get creative with massage, oral, sensation play and toys. When a penis isn't as erect as you want it to be, ask yourself: *What is possible, exciting and pleasurable right now?*

✳ Remember you can have a lot of fun with a soft cock. Penises can give and receive a lot of pleasure when they're soft. Explore new sensations like cupping the balls or the shaft – or if you're having sex with someone, sucking the shaft, dry humping or thrusting. You do not need to be hard to have a good time.

✳ Seek professional support. If it's affecting you, it may be worthwhile seeking individual support.

PREMATURE EJACULATION

Premature ejaculation (PE) is a common condition. Various studies have found that between 20 to 30 per cent of men experience it, but it is likely underreported. It's characterised by an inability to delay climax, or ejaculation that occurs in one minute or less. People often have different ideas of what cumming 'too quickly' means. For some, it's finishing within seconds of penetration, while for others, five minutes can feel short.

It's important to see a GP for an assessment, especially if you notice a sudden change in how long you can last. The causes could be genetic, other health problems such as abnormal hormonal levels, or psychosocial issues like stress, anxiety, confidence or relationship issues. Treatments for PE will vary based on whether it is a lifelong concern (i.e. it's been a concern since your first or early sexual experiences) or if it's acquired later in life. When you're affected by PE, it can feel really stressful, but the good news is: there's so much you can do to regain control over when you climax. With some basic at-home practices, you'll see results really quickly. Here are a few foundational tools.

Awareness and regulation

In most cases, people with PE are so unaware that their arousal is building that they don't know they're cumming until they're actually cumming. This limits their ability to control their orgasm and shortens their pleasure experience. I help my clients bring mindfulness to their body, helping them tune in to sensory cues to monitor, assess and calm their arousal system.

As a starting point, try the following body scan.

1. Find a comfortable position where you feel at ease.

2. Take a few deep, mindful breaths.

3. Starting at your toes, move your focus slowly through your body in an upwards direction, paying attention to each sensation in your feet, calves, knees, thighs, hips and so on …

4. When your attention wanders, gently return back to your body scan, pausing on any part that feels particularly pleasurable.

5. Once you've reached the top of your head, take in your body as a whole, noticing any emotions that arise.

6. Take another moment for a few deep breaths, releasing any tension as you exhale.

Regulation is a useful practice for lengthening your experience. By learning to up-regulate and down-regulate your arousal, you'll be better able to control it. Breath is a simple but effective tool to help you last longer, as it works to reduce stress and activate your parasympathetic nervous system, often referred to as the rest-and-digest system. When it comes to lasting longer, you want to be in your calm state. Practise down-regulating breath every day by using the simple box breathing technique described in Chapter 2 to down-regulate arousal in and out of sex.

Arousal ladder

My PE clients are *always* early to every session – a few have even turned up a week early, thinking their session was that day. They are premature with many aspects of life; they move through it at a fast pace.

The way we think has a direct impact on how much sensation we feel and how we can regulate arousal in the body, and it can also impact sexual ability. People who struggle with premature ejaculation can feel such a crippling sense of anxiety and pressure to perform that the sense of not being good enough becomes a self-fulfilling prophecy. They're so disconnected from their body, so stressed that they're going to cum immediately, that sure enough, they cum immediately. We need to rebuild confidence, and one way to do that is through practice.

I start by teaching them about the arousal ladder, where 0 is not aroused, 9 is the point of no return, and 10 is orgasm. We always practise this awareness outside of a sexual context first, to make it easier to apply during sex. We then apply it to a four-week masturbation program (see overleaf).

The Arousal Ladder

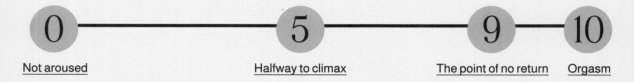

0	5	9	10
Not aroused	Halfway to climax	The point of no return	Orgasm

The four-week masturbation program

This is all about bringing awareness to your body and finding ways to build arousal. The aim is to practise awareness and regulation in masturbation – it's not about maintaining an erection, nor is it about orgasm. Set a timer for 5 to 10 minutes. Aim to repeat each step a few times and practise a few times a week.

Week one: Build arousal with masturbation to a 5 out of 10, then take hands off and down-regulate arousal to about a 1. Repeat until the timer goes off.

Week two: Build arousal with masturbation to a 6, then keep hands on but stop moving them and down-regulate arousal to about a 3. Repeat until the timer goes off.

Week three: Build arousal with masturbation to a 7, then keep hands on but this time keep moving and slowing the touch to down-regulate arousal to about a 5. Include movement, breath, placement of awareness and/or touch. Repeat until the timer goes off.

Week four: Build arousal with masturbation to an 8, then this time engage your pelvic floor muscles (the muscles you engage to stop yourself from peeing) for a few rounds of breath. Keep hands on but this time keep moving and slowing the touch to down-regulate arousal to about a 5. Include movement, breath, placement of awareness and/or touch. Repeat until the timer goes off.

Add levels of difficulty. You could try toys, pelvic floor exercises, certain positions that you know to be more challenging, or even inviting a partner into the practice session with you. (I know this can feel vulnerable, but it's likely your partner wants to help!)

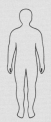

Pelvic floor exercises

A consistent pelvic floor practice strengthens your pubococcygeus (PC) muscle, which can be useful in addressing many sexual concerns. Awareness of your PC can help delay or control ejaculation in the same way it helps you stop yourself from peeing – you engage your PC muscles before you ejaculate. A study found that 82 per cent of men who suffered lifelong premature ejaculation were able to last longer after 12 weeks of pelvic floor exercises – a pretty impressive result for this humble practice. Pelvic floor exercises are useful for all people as they can also support you in becoming more aware of your body, being able to regulate arousal, and feeling more pleasure and sensation. They are certainly worth practising.

1. Start with the basics. When you next go to pee, do a pelvic floor contraction just before you let go, aiming to hold the contraction for a few seconds. This is a really low-effort way to integrate pelvic floor exercises into your life.

2. Try to do two sets of these contractions twice a day when you pee for the next two weeks, making note of any differences in your arousal or ejaculation control.

3. Some people choose to do them every time they stop at a traffic light. You may set a daily timer – or even better, practise squeezing and releasing your pelvic floor while masturbating.

There are a few key ways you can strengthen your pelvic floor muscles: speed, duration, intensity and reverse.

✳ Speed = how many you can pump out in a designated time.

✳ Duration = how long you hold each rep for.

✳ Intensity = the force (intensity) at which you engage your pelvic floor.

✳ Reverse = the release rather than the engagement of PC muscles.

It is worth noting that pelvic floor exercises aren't for everyone. If you have a vagina and penetration is painful, uncomfortable or not possible, I'd recommend booking in with a pelvic health physio for diagnosis and treatment options.

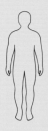

Orgasm multiple times

While multiple orgasms don't need to be saved for solo sex, there is a lot we can learn from masturbation in applying it to sex. Having multiple orgasms can be an intensely pleasurable experience (obviously). Here are some general things you can try to build up pleasure and get yourself (or your partner) on course for experiencing multiple orgasms:

* Take your time to build arousal.

* Try using your breath, moving gently, incorporating sounds and touch, and even taking the time to consciously direct your mental awareness towards other parts of your body.

* Practise pelvic floor exercises – engage and release your pelvic floor.

* Try edging – bring yourself to the point of orgasm, but stop just before you're about to cum. Then allow yourself to relax before repeating. You can do this any number of times, and it really helps to increase orgasm intensity and amount.

* Have your toys and lubes ready – their sole function is to make sex feel great.

Redefine sex

Draw a circle and inside it write all the things that sex can be to you. Include actions, emotions and intentions. This is your new definition of sex, one that reflects your curiosities and interests. Any time you feel hung-up on orgasm, come back to your circle and check you're not pursuing orgasm in a heteronormative way. It's kinda puritanical to assume that anything other than penis in vagina isn't 'natural' and it can limit how much pleasure we can access during sex.

IMPORTANT STUFF

✳ While orgasms are a big part of sex, they're not the only part. Being goal focused will add to the stress – it's important to ease any pressure or stress you feel to perform.

✳ Find different ways to end sex – a great sexual experience does not always end in orgasm. Maybe set a timer and that's when you stop having sex, or take breaks throughout.

✳ Pre-orgasmia, erectile dysfunction and premature ejaculation are really common, and can be overcome. As a starting point, it's important to see a GP to rule out any health issues.

✳ Building arousal and experiencing orgasm is possible, though it takes practice to build awareness of pleasure and sensation in your body. Start with regular solo sex practice.

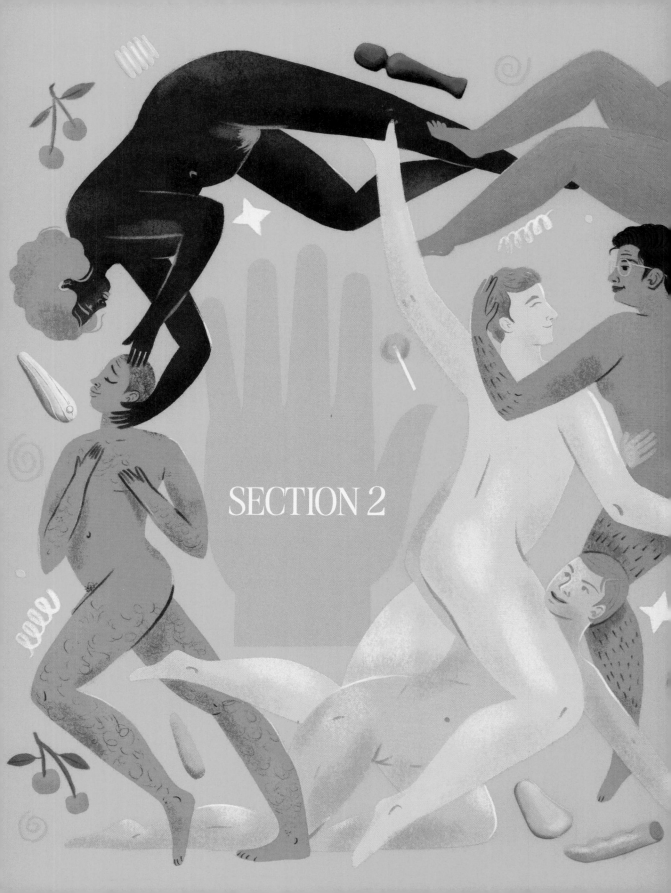

SECTION 2

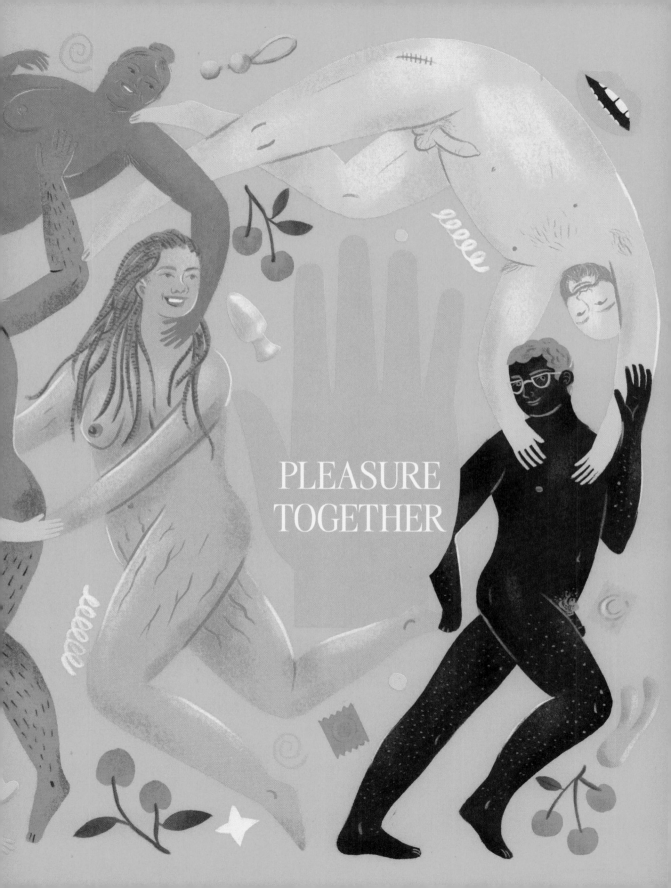

PLEASURE
TOGETHER

BOUNDARIES AND CONSENT

How do I talk about consent without killing the mood? How do I let my sexual partner(s) know I'm no longer into it? How can I advocate for myself without making them feel bad? How can I be open to hearing no when I feel rejected? In this chapter we cover consent – arguably the most important sex skill.

In a time when open and nuanced discussion about consent is, unfortunately, new to the mainstream, there's a lot we need to relearn. We often frame consent as something we need to teach in order to prevent bad things happening, which is obviously really important – but it's the bare minimum. Consent is about actively discussing boundaries to make sure everyone has the best possible experience.

In this conversation with our words and bodies, we can all become better partners. I don't say this lightly: if you want to be a good lover, fuck the fingering techniques and positions and learn about consent.

These principles apply whether you're having a one-night stand or are in a ten-year relationship. Every single time we have sex, we need to be actively engaged with consent so that we can, as writer Jaclyn Friedman so perfectly states, 'have sex in a way that leaves everyone involved feeling more fully human, not less'. We all have the capacity to violate someone else's boundaries, and we all have the capacity to make someone feel comfortable and safe.

Unlike what we're often told, consent doesn't have to feel confusing, offensive or be a buzz kill. When I talk to people about the topics of consent and boundaries, I hear a few common concerns:

✳ 'Speaking about sex and checking in kills the mood.'

✳ 'Consent can feel confusing.'

✳ 'I don't know how to share my boundaries without offending someone.'

I'm frustrated every time someone says, *I'm worried it'll kill the mood*. Not necessarily frustrated with the person, but with the systems at large that have made us think good sex is seamless, like sex in a movie: two people bust open an apartment door, hands ferociously moving over every body part, ripping clothes off; they can't even make it to the bedroom before they both cum at the same time then fall in a satisfied heap on the floor. Sure, this looks hot in a movie, but it teaches us nothing about consent. Where's the talking? The checking in? The safer-sex practices? Where's the lube?!

If you feel it's too awkward to have a conversation about consent before sex, ask yourself: *Where did I learn this?* Where did you hear this *first*? I find it interesting that talking about consent is what most people say is the most awkward part – not the getting naked, exchanging bodily fluids, rubbing genitals together, and not the idea that we may be doing something that the other person doesn't like. If you find talking about consent clunky, you are human. But this is a non-negotiable when it comes to sex. If there's no consent, there is no mood. Consent is about making sure everyone has the best possible experience. If one person is uncomfortable, they're unlikely to leave feeling more fully human.

🖐 97

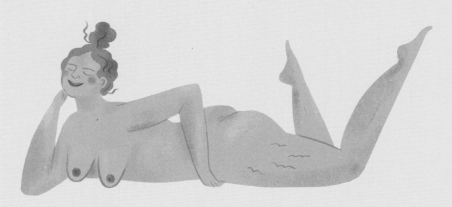

MY DEFINITION OF CONSENT

When I talk about consent, I'm referring to both the verbal and nonverbal communication that ensures everyone involved is willing and excited to be there. Because I mean, isn't that what you want? Consent means freely saying yes to sexual experiences and being able to stop, slow down or pause at any time. It's communicating with others to ensure you have the best sexual experience possible. Consent is specific (consenting to one thing doesn't mean you've consented to anything else) and consenting to something once doesn't mean you've promised to do it again, even if you are in a relationship with someone. It's not consent if someone has been drinking heavily or taking drugs, is a minor, or is being pressured or coerced into anything. Without consent, you are not having sex: that is rape.

In recent years we've seen affirmative consent legislated into a few Australian states. I hope that sentence dates really quickly and that by the time you read this it is law in every state. Affirmative consent places the responsibility on every individual involved to actively communicate and check that the others involved are also consenting. It moves away from the 'no means no' rhetoric we all grew up with and instead emphasises 'yes means yes'. It centres active and ongoing communication. Instead of blaming the victim with rhetoric like 'They didn't say no', we ask, 'Did you seek a yes?'

The legal definition of affirmative consent states that consent is never assumed, it requires ongoing verbal and nonverbal communication, and must be freely and voluntarily given. In her book *Consent Laid Bare*, Chanel Contos states, 'As a legal reform, this is monumental, as the onus is on the accused to prove they sought and received consent. Affirmative consent laws aim to shift the blame from the victim to the perpetrator by encouraging people to actively seek consent.'

Affirmative consent also accounts for the freeze or fawn response. (If you need a reminder about how this works, see the section on sex and stress in Chapter 2.) Freezing in the face of a threat may mean someone doesn't actively push someone away, or say 'no', as they may be unable to formulate sentences, stay present or communicate. This does not mean they are consenting. Fawning is also a response in threat of danger where the victim tries to appease the aggressor in order to survive the danger. As a fellow fawner, I am familiar with how confusing this response can be. I've found myself asking, *Why was I nice to that person who was inflicting harm – why didn't I run away or tell them to fuck off?* Fawn responses are common. In the moment of danger, it feels like the only option is to appease the aggressor in order to stay safe.

FIGURING OUT YOUR BOUNDARIES

It's true that sometimes we don't recognise a boundary until we've met it. Our boundaries may surprise us too. *Huh, I thought I'd be into that but it turns out it didn't feel great.* Understanding our boundaries is another classic case of learning by doing. But we can still spend time reflecting on what may be a *yes, no, maybe* or *I need more information.* This may start with research or a conversation with a friend. At times you may even have a pretty clear somatic response (i.e. your body responds before your rational thought).

To explore your boundaries, feel into how your body responds to the list of sexual acts on the next page – as you read them, take a breath; does it feel like a *yes, no, maybe* or *I need more information*? (You can also apply this to the much longer list at the end of this book.)

Kissing

Anal

Dry
humping

Scissoring

Fingering

Masturbation

Oral

Flirting

First dates

Toys

Sensual
massage

Spanking

Power
play

Dirty talk

Fucking

Group
sex

Role
play

How did your body respond? Start trying to identify what you want, like and need. You may want to expand on this research by observing how you respond to the different sexual acts described in this book, or by exploring fantasies while you masturbate, watching ethical porn, talking with friends, and reading erotica. It could be as simple as taking a few moments to feel into it – what does my body want?

Talking about consent with non-sexual partners is fundamental in establishing a felt sense of our own boundaries. It also illuminates ideas in us. Being exposed to new ways of thinking can help us get a sense of what we're into, and speaking openly about sex with others connects us, validates us and equips us with information, and it disrupts the oppressive sentiment that consent must be quiet and unspoken.

CREATING SPACE

Some things are easier to say than others. You might find that asking 'How does this feel?' or 'What would make this better?' is a lot easier than 'How would you like to be touched?' No matter how you say it, checking in during sex is valuable,

important, and will probably mean you're having better sex too. Chapter 8 contains heaps of prompts for you – sometimes it helps to have a few ideas as starting points.

The signals we send to each other – verbal and nonverbal – can either create space for someone to express a boundary or can create an implicit pressure to comply. Ask yourself: *Am I setting up an environment for consensual interactions, or one that risks coercion?*

Here are some ways you create an environment for consensual interactions:

✳ Demonstrate that you're listening and respecting boundaries in non-sexual contexts. For example, if you're on a date and someone tells you they want a non-alcoholic drink, don't try to convince them to get a beer or belittle them for their choice. If they say they don't want to talk about a particular topic, don't dig deeper. If someone pulls away when you touch them – even something like trying to hold hands – take it as a no and let them make the next move towards physical contact. If you haven't kissed someone before, instead of awkwardly leaning in, mouth open, why don't you try saying, 'Can I kiss you?' or 'I really want to kiss you' and wait for their response.

* Pay attention to verbal and nonverbal consent signals before and during sex. Some people find it challenging to say an explicit and unambiguous no out loud. Nonverbal cues are really important for those who feel they lose their voice or don't know what to say, or for those who feel their voice/mouth is restrained or compromised. When it comes to nonverbal consent, try something as simple as holding up your hands in a stop signal.

* Tune in to the other person. If you're having sex with someone and they look disconnected, disassociated or as though they're not experiencing a full-body yes, that's when you need to take the initiative to check in with them and ensure everything is still okay. How is this for you? Do you want to do things differently? What would make it better? Learn to read and respect a nonverbal no.

* Abide by the agreements you made. Even if sex is moving quickly and passionately, by abiding by your agreement, you're showing them you've understood, and that you respect their consent.

* If there is a 'no', an 'I'm not sure', or a pause – *stop immediately*. Not another thrust, kiss, touch or lick. Stop immediately and check in. This creates the context for consent to be comfortably expressed and to be heard.

* You can change your mind, and you must allow space for others to change their minds too. Just because it excited you at one point, or you agreed to one thing, doesn't mean you've said an ongoing yes or a yes to everything. This understanding also fosters space for creativity and curiosity, knowing that you can try something and if you don't like it you don't have to go through with it.

'BLUE BALLS' AS SEXUAL COERCION

The phrase 'blue balls' is used to describe the discomfort experienced when an erection lasts for a period of time without orgasm. When you're aroused, blood flow to the genitals is increased. This is known as epididymal hypertension, and can feel like aching, heaviness or discomfort in the testicles. Despite the name 'blue balls', testicles typically won't turn blue, and it usually isn't serious.

While it may be uncomfortable, blue balls are not dangerous, and any discomfort should pass when arousal decreases. The key here is: it's no one else's responsibility to relieve this discomfort. We all have erectile tissue in our genitals, so all people can experience a sense of discomfort from being sexually aroused without release, but we very rarely hear about 'blue vulva'. Cis men are socialised by media, pornography and general society to expect someone to satisfy them. Cis women or people with vulvas can also experience a sense of discomfort if they are aroused for an extended period of time without the release of climax. However, they are socialised to expect, self-manage or cope with sexual discomfort.

Using 'blue balls' to guilt someone into starting or continuing sexual activity is an example of sexual coercion. Sexual coercion is unwanted sexual activity that happens when you are pressured, tricked, threatened or forced in a non-physical way. Trying to argue or guilt-trip someone into sex is not consent; it is sex without consent, which is assault. Remember: consent is reversible, which means it can be revoked at any time.

HOW TO MANAGE BLUE BALLS ON YOUR OWN

* Masturbate.
* Take some time, rest and the arousal will subside.
* Read a book, listen to a podcast, distract yourself by thinking about something non-sexual.
* Make a cup of tea, drink it together.
* Watch a show.
* Do some high-intensity exercise.
* Have a shower.
* Lengthen your exhale.
* And remind yourself: no one ever owes sex to you. You never owe sex to anyone.

WHEN SOMEONE SAYS NO

We need to talk about how it feels to hear 'no'. It can suck! It can hurt! Especially if you've felt vulnerable asking for what you need, or if you really like the person. But no matter how much it hurts, you have no right to violate that boundary, pressure the person to change their mind, or coerce them into giving you what you want.

Here's a better approach to dealing with a 'no': don't take it personally.

If someone isn't into you or something you want, instead of taking it personally or going on the attack, say thank you.

THE NO GAME

Play this with anyone – a lover, family member, friend, therapist. One person feels into any request they'd like to make. This could be anything: *Can I have a hug*? *Will you kiss my forehead*? *May I touch your arms*? *Can I have a blanket*? *I want you to hold me* ... And then the other person says no. And then the first person says thank you, and then keeps making requests, to which the other person keeps saying no. After a few minutes of this game, discuss. What did you notice?

This can be revealing, intense, interesting and absurd. Once you've played a few rounds, instead of just no, the responses can be *yes, no* or *can I have more information?* Observe how your body responds. How does it feel when you say yes to something that feels like it should be a no? How does it feel to endure or place others' needs above your own? When you're finished, discuss what you've learnt.

That could sound like:

✳ 'Thanks for letting me know, it's great to know where you're at.'

✳ 'Thanks. If you're not into it, I don't want to do it.'

✳ 'Thanks for telling me you're not into that. Is there something else that you'd like to do instead?'

Saying thank you shows that you respect their boundaries and openness. It communicates that you've heard them, and it also helps you see the boundary as a useful piece of information rather than a rejection.

It can also be helpful to process your response with some solo enquiry. You might choose to write about it, discuss it with a friend or get some professional support. Find ways to support yourself to ensure you don't make others feel responsible for saying no.

SENDING NUDES

Consent is essential when sending and receiving nude pics. Have an open conversation and make sure you ascertain written or verbal consent. Here are some ways you can seek consent before sending nudes. I have framed these questions for those who have established a safe and consensual relationship. (Please note: these are not to be confused with an opening liner on a dating app – that is rarely ever okay.)

* I want to send you a pic of what I'm not wearing ;) Do you want to see it?

* I think it'd be really (fire emoji) if we sent each other nudes someday. Would you be into that?

* I'm feeling good today. Can I show you?

* How do you feel about sending nudes?

* If we ever were to send nudes, what agreements can we make to ensure we feel safe?

* I'm naked, wanna see?

Once you're ready to take a pic, consider playing music that makes you feel comfortable or sexy, using props like fabric to conceal and reveal, and focusing on areas of your body that you love. People are pretty quick to jump to full-frontal dick pics, but that is just the TIP of the iceberg. Sometimes less is more. Start with a bit of leg, lower back, stomach, underwear or breast/chest, and build up from there. You could try using a mirror to get the angle you want, moving or swaying while taking a pic or only partially exposing yourself at first. Perhaps you would feel more comfortable in your favourite underwear? Or in a really bubbly bath? The only rules are the ones you make.

Continue to check in after you've sent the pic. Does it still feel good/exciting? What could make the experience feel even better?

A NOTE ON SAFETY AND SECURITY

Before sending any nudes, ensure you've established a clear agreement. Where are you sending the photos? Do you create a private thread? Is there a time of day that's more appropriate? Will they be saved or deleted? How will you keep them secure and private? What agreements or boundaries do you want to set? Sharing intimate images without consent is a criminal offence. This is called 'image-based abuse' and is criminalised at state and federal levels.

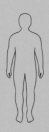

The Three-minute Game

Communication is a two-way street that requires you to hold space for others. Everyone involved has a responsibility to find their communication style. Every single person who has sex should play the Three-minute Game, and revisit it constantly. It is a simple yet powerful resource created by life coach Harry Faddis and further developed by Dr Betty Martin, a certified sex educator and coach, who is a pioneer in the field of sexology and human relationships.

This is a game I set for most couples for at-home practice, as a way to establish communication, consent and boundaries. I know not everyone is going to play this before a one-night stand, but I think it would make all sexual experiences one squillion times better.

You'll need a comfortable space and a timer set to three-minute increments. Dedicate at least 30 minutes to this exercise. Consent is the foundation of this game. Check in with your body and what you want/need. Decide who is Person A and who is Person B.

Person A asks:

1. 'How would you like to be touched for three minutes?' Communicate, discuss boundaries and consent, then once you're clear on what's going to happen, you have up to three minutes to do the touch, and you can change your mind at any time.

2. 'How would you like to touch me for three minutes?' Communicate, discuss boundaries and consent, then once you're clear on what's going to happen, you have up to three minutes to do the touch, and you can change your mind at any time.

Then swap and Person B asks those questions.

Each of the four rounds of the game creates a different role for you:

✳ Serve: you are doing and it's for them.

✳ Take: you are doing and it's for you.

✳ Accept: they are doing and it's for you.

✳ Allow: they are doing and it's for them.

Each round may challenge you in different ways and hopefully be enjoyable, probably in different ways as well. The point is to distinguish between the different roles you're experiencing. Ask yourself: *Who is this for?* Go slowly, start with short turns and neutral body areas. Start playing this game in a non-sexual way, clothes on. Then you may want to start exploring erogenous zones and making the game more sexual as you go.

THE WHEEL OF CONSENT

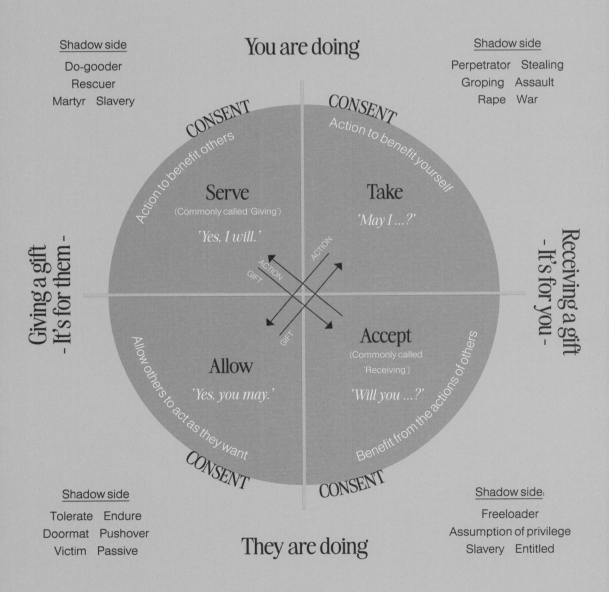

Shadow side
Do-gooder
Rescuer
Martyr   Slavery

You are doing

Shadow side
Perpetrator   Stealing
Groping   Assault
Rape   War

CONSENT
Action to benefit others

CONSENT
Action to benefit yourself

Giving a gift
- It's for them -

Serve
(Commonly called 'Giving')

'Yes, I will.'

Take

'May I …?'

Receiving a gift
- It's for you -

ACTION

ACTION

GIFT

GIFT

Allow

'Yes, you may.'

Accept
(Commonly called 'Receiving')

'Will you …?'

Allow others to act as they want

Benefit from the actions of others

CONSENT

CONSENT

Shadow side
Tolerate   Endure
Doormat   Pushover
Victim   Passive

They are doing

Shadow side:
Freeloader
Assumption of privilege
Slavery   Entitled

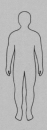

The Wheel of Consent

Dr Betty Martin has been developing and teaching the Wheel of Consent for around 15 years. This is an approach to learning consent through your body; it explores the dynamics of 'receiving' and 'giving', knowing what you want, and being able to communicate this with others.

If you haven't already played the Three-minute Game, I recommend you do so before working through this next part. It will make more sense once you've practised the game – as Betty Martin says, 'It's the experience of it that will change you.'

In any instance of touch, there are two factors: who's doing it and who it's for. Those two factors combine in four ways, represented in the illustration on the previous page in four quadrants. Each quadrant presents its own challenges, lessons and joys. You may feel like you spend more of your life and your sexual experiences with one quadrant, and there may be others you wish to practise. Serving, Accepting, Taking and Allowing are all important for a healthy and sensual relationship, so long as they are practised consensually. Anytime you are outside of consent, they are no longer useful. The circle represents consent (which is your agreement). Inside the circle, there is a gift given and a gift received. Outside the circle (which is without your consent), the same action becomes stealing, abusing and so on.

There's a lot going on here, so let's break it down.

Serving quadrant

When you are doing and it's for them, we call this 'serving'. You've already practised this quadrant when you played the Three-minute Game and you asked: 'How do you want to be touched?'

When you are serving, you:

1. Set aside what you prefer (including the response you hope to see).

2. Ask what your partner wants – and wait for the answer. Making space for their choice is the most important part.

3. Decide if you are willing and able to do that. Honour your limits. Ask yourself: *Is this something I can give with a full heart?* If it is, do so as best you can.

4. Say you're welcome!

You contribute to their experience. The gift you give is your action. So essentially, you are doing something for the benefit of others.

Accepting quadrant

When you are being touched and it's for your enjoyment we call this 'accepting'. You've already practised this quadrant when you played the Three-minute Game and your partner asked you: 'How do you want to be touched?'

When you are accepting, you:

1. Put yourself first. Set aside what you are just okay with. Go for wonderful.

2. Take all the time you need to notice what it is you would like. This is the most important part, and often the hardest.

3. Ask as directly and specifically as you can. No hinting, no maybes, no 'whatever you want to give'.

4. Stop trying to 'give' your giver a good experience. That's their job.

5. Can change your mind any time (and ask for something different).

6. Say thank you!

So essentially, you are receiving a gift from the actions of others.

Taking quadrant

When you are doing something and it is for your own enjoyment, instead of your partner's enjoyment, we call this 'taking'. You've already practised this quadrant when you played the Three-minute Game and you responded to the question: 'How would you like to touch me?' This is hard for almost everyone, and often feels odd, elusive or scary. Taking is receiving the gift of access. In order to receive this gift, you must stop trying to 'give'.

When you are taking, you:

1. Ask your partner what their limits are and abide by them, completely.

2. Take the time to notice what part of them you would like to feel.

3. Ask 'May I …' not 'Would you like …'

4. Use your hands to feel, not to serve. Move slowly; the slower you go, the more you feel. Feel for the shape and texture.

5. Remember – if you start trying to give to them – this touch is for you.

6. Say thank you!

Essentially, you are taking action for your own benefit.

Allowing quadrant

When you are being touched and it is for the enjoyment of the other person, we call this 'allowing'. You've already practised this quadrant when you played the Three-minute Game and you asked: 'How would you like to touch me?' This is very easy for some, very hard for others. It depends on knowing you have a choice about how you are touched. Allowing is a form of giving. The gift you give is access to you. Set aside what you would prefer. Take responsibility for your limits.

When you are allowing, you:

1. Take the time to consider your limits. Ask yourself: *Is this a gift I can give with a full heart?*

2. Wait for a resounding inner 'Yes!' If you are hesitant, it's one of these:

   a) You need more information.

   b) It's a no waiting for you to hear it.

   c) If you set a certain limit, it would be a yes; ask yourself what that limit is.

3. Say you're welcome!

Essentially, you're allowing others to take action, while keeping your own limits.

I know that's a lot to digest! For a more extensive tutorial, please visit Betty Martin's website, and read her book (written with Robyn Dalzen), *The Art of Receiving and Giving: The Wheel of Consent*.

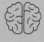
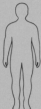

Yes, no, can I have more information?

This game requires two people and is about asking questions and creating space for the answer. You're not required to actually act out any requests. After you've played it a few times you may want to add the option to do the touch.

Decide who is person A and who is person B.

✳ Person A, ask for anything you want. Take your time, breathe, resist the urge to rush.

✳ Person B, resist the urge to answer straight away. Take a breath, feel into how your body responds to the request. Once you have a sense of your answer, you can say *yes*, *no* or *can I have more information?*

✳ Person A, if B said *yes* or *no*, your response to them will be *thank you*. If they said, *can I have more information?* describe your request in detail.

✳ Repeat for 5 minutes, then switch roles.

✳ Discuss the experience with each other: *What was that like for you?*

IMPORTANT STUFF

✳ Consent is essential and an incredibly valuable life skill in terms of communication, observing emotions and learning how to check in.

✳ If you find it hard to have conversations around consent, I'd recommend really asking yourself why that's the case. Practise it, make it part of your day-to-day relationships, and you'll notice it becomes more integrated.

✳ Whether you're practising verbal or nonverbal consent, remember that sex without consent isn't sex; it's rape.

✳ Consent makes sex hot and pleasurable for everyone involved.

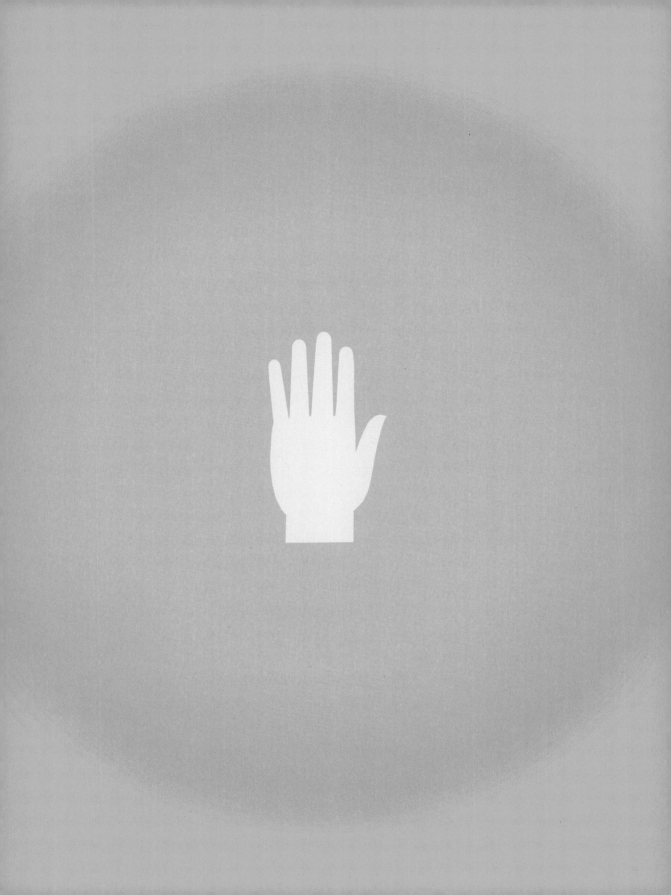

SEXUAL COMMUNICATION

How will you get what you want if you can't even talk about it? Talking about sex is like learning a whole new language – it is as much about identifying what you want as it is about communicating it. In this chapter, we'll cover the foundations of how to talk about sex (yes, even the most awkward conversations), learn some practical communication tools and work through a few exercises to put it into practice.

What do you want? It's a question that seems to derail most of us, even those who see themselves as confident, self-assured, sexual people who *know* that no one is a mind reader. When someone asks you what you want, they're probably really curious about your body, needs and desires.

They probably want more information in order to help you feel really good, or maybe they want to check in to make sure you're really into something. They also may feel a little lost and need direction. Plus, for many, it can be a real turn-on hearing what their partner likes.

But this question can feel terrifying because it holds so much meaning and can feel so revealing. We might go into a panicked spiral: *I don't know what I want! Whatever you're doing is fine? I actually do know what I want, but am I allowed to ask that? If I ask for that, will they be able to do it? What if they try to do it but it doesn't feel as good as I hoped it would? And what does it say about me that I want this? Is this a weird or gross thing to ask for? Is this normal?* Instead of answering, we might freeze, or say 'I don't know', or endure something we're not really into.

Sexual communication is the verbal and nonverbal way we connect with others to check in, build arousal and ultimately make sure everyone is having a good time and getting what they want. I constantly see how good sexual communication skills can solve most sex-related concerns and can help all people get closer to having fulfilling sex. It can feel challenging to ask for what you want, especially if

you're new to sex talk, and because it feels daunting at first, it's all too common to shut down and avoid the clunkiness. So before working on what to say, we need to address why you're not talking.

Let's add some perspective. Imagine you and your sexual partner are in a new kitchen. You've never been there before. You've got to make dinner together, but you're not allowed to speak. You have no idea what the other person feels like eating, or when they want to eat – you don't even know if they're hungry. But you both have to start cooking. You don't know where the pots and pans are either, or where the good oil is kept. You're pulling out drawers, trying to suss out their reactions to what you're making, trying to gauge if they're into this meal and just kinda hoping they'll like what you come up with. This is how most people have sex.

Talking about what you want often starts with learning about what you want. I've noticed that for a lot of my clients, the fear of not knowing exactly what they want is the thing that stops them from even trying. Knowing what you need is a process – you will always be learning. It's less about communicating the exact technique or style of sex or exactly how you want to be touched, kissed or sucked. Instead, I'd say it's more a process of acknowledging we won't know straight away; we need to pause to feel into it. Knowing what you want is about feeling, communicating, experimenting, and being non-attached to the goal of sex and following what feels good.

Have you ever desperately wanted to speak about something but felt terrified it'll offend the other person or make them retreat more? Yeah, same – and I've literally spent years learning how to talk about sex. When we want to talk about something that feels risky, it's as though the words are on the tip of the tongue but we have no idea how to actually say them.

I want to introduce you to a phrase I use with my clients who feel stuck. I invite them to say this to themselves and each other before having an edgy conversation.

We're here to do things differently.

I love working with this phrase. Any time you feel stuck, nervous, uninspired or awkward, remember: you're intending to do things differently. It may take some time, and it certainly may be a little clunky (because you'll want to revert to what you know!). However, that's a sign that you're at your 'learning edge'.

WHY DON'T WE ASK FOR WHAT WE WANT?

Fear of rejection. Judgement. Not knowing how to ask. Not knowing what I want. Shame. Anticipating they will say no. Systems of oppression make me feel undeserving. Keeping status quo. Conditioning. In case it's used against me. Disgusted by my body. It feels too risky. It may not be as good as I expect. Don't believe it's possible. Feels pointless; it's never good. I might actually get it. Disconnected from body. Power dynamic imbalance. It's easier to do it myself. Feeling unworthy. Having to reciprocate. Punishment (by myself or other). Unwanted consequences. Too hard. Too vulnerable. Expecting them to know what I want. Tired of asking. Fear of violence. Guilt. Body shaming. Stigma. Feeling I don't deserve pleasure until I earn it. Told I might not be allowed. Believing the need is wrong. Kink shaming. Slut shaming. Taboo. Performance anxiety. No exposure to people voicing needs. Wanting to be low-maintenance. People-pleasing tendencies. Lack of resources. Low self-esteem. Isolation. Socialisation. Low confidence. Upbringing. Biases. Anticipated discomfort. Trauma.

TALK ABOUT IT FIRST OUTSIDE OF SEX

When first bringing up a sexual concern or curiosity, try starting the conversation outside of a sexual context – so, not directly before, during or after sex. The main reason for this is that these times can feel particularly vulnerable, and you may not be in the ideal state to have a conversation. Find a time that is free from distraction – you might be on a walk or out at dinner or having down time together.

A conversation starter may sound like:

✳ 'I love having sex with you and I'd like to talk about how we could make it even better. When suits you?'

✳ 'As you know, sex is really important to me. I'm hoping we could speak about what we like, don't like and what we want to explore. What do you think?'

✳ 'I'm reading this book about sex and there's a whole chapter on communication, and I realised we don't really speak about sex. Do you want to go through some of the practices with me?'

TALKING DURING SEX

Talking during sex is useful for endless reasons. It helps us check in and get the right touch, and it can turn us on and keep us present. We've discussed the importance of talking outside of sex, which is a process I take my clients through too. We must first address why we're not talking, identify what is pleasurable, then practise talking outside of sex. It would be totally unrealistic to give you a few one-liners and say, 'Go on, use this exact sentence to get what you want every time' and expect you to feel equipped to do so. (Although don't worry, at the end of this chapter I'll give you over 50 one-liners to try, because when we're learning a new language it's so useful to get examples!)

Start simply, with verbal communication cues such as 'I like that' or 'I'd love it if you did this'. Also practise nonverbal communication, like touch, eye contact, sounds, and gesturing with your body.

This is often easier said than done, and in moments when you're lost for words I know it can be useful to turn to a guide. I learnt the following process from Dr Betty Martin. I recommend trying this outside of a sexual context first.

How to communicate a need or desire

✳ **Notice:** What do I want? A specific kind of touch, an opportunity to be held, some alone time? This is the practice of regularly bringing awareness to your body and noticing your needs.

✳ **Trust:** Believe the impulse. Trust your body and its needs.

✳ **Value:** See value in your needs and yourself as an erotic person, worthy of pleasure.

✳ **Communicate:** Request and allow for a response.

How to respond when someone communicates a need or desire

✳ **Notice:** Notice your limits. Are you willing or comfortable with their request?

✳ **Trust:** Believe your impulse. How does your body feel upon hearing their need or desire? Can you lean into trusting your response? Is it a 'Hell yeah!', 'not sure', 'no thanks', or 'I'd love to know a little more'?

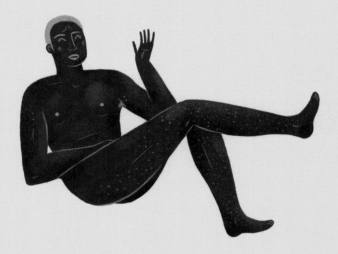

✳ **Value:** Value your limits. Does the request exist within your boundaries? For example, you may feel comfortable with someone touching your face but not your hair.

✳ **Communicate:** Be as direct, clear and descriptive as you can, to let them know exactly what you are and aren't willing to do.

LEARNING TO RECEIVE

I think all people will really benefit from unpacking the idea of 'receiving'. A lot of people really struggle with this. When all the attention is on your pleasure and genitals, the noise in your head can take you out of your body and out of the moment, limiting your pleasure and your ability to feel anything, and often resulting in a spike in anxiety. More often than not, the first thing we need to do is talk about it. When clients struggle with this, I'll often ask them, 'What is getting in the way of you being comfortable with receiving?' Some common themes include: self-consciousness, body confidence, performance anxiety, not feeling deserving of pleasure, a history of trauma, childbirth, or a combination of these things. If it's really affecting you and your relationship, you may find it helpful to speak to a trusted health professional or a loved one about your concerns.

A LITTLE REASSURANCE CAN GO A LONG WAY

When you speak about your concerns with a partner and ask for reassurance, it can create space for you both to feel more comfortable, reassured and validated. You could try any of the following:

✳ 'I struggle to stay present because I'm worried you're uncomfortable. Will you tell me if you ever need to pause?'

✳ 'I find it really edgy/vulnerable when you go down on me because I worry about [insert reason here]. Can we work on this together?'

✳ 'It'll really help me receive if you tell me what you like about giving.'

While this can feel like a solo journey, you don't have to struggle through distraction on your own. So often my clients will tell me they want to be more present or they want to support their partner in feeling more present – often there's a lot we can do together to feel more relaxed and present while giving and receiving. For more information on learning to be present, refer back to Chapter 2.

SUPPORTING A PARTNER TO RECEIVE

For most people, knowing their partner enjoys touching their body and giving them pleasure is an important precursor to fully releasing into the moment. With clear, affirmative language, remind your partner what you love about touching, kissing or going down on them. Remind them that you've got the time, space and energy to give, and that if you need a break, you'll tell them.

In a session I once had with a heterosexual couple, the wife said, 'I just want to know that you like going down on me.' Her husband responded, 'Yeah, I don't mind it.' In that moment, I could see her whole body sink. She was shattered and took his lack of enthusiasm as proof that she was unwanted, too needy and not sexy. After spending time with his response, we learnt that he actually did love going down on her, he just didn't have the language to voice it. He didn't know whether it would be creepy or inappropriate to enjoy it so much, even though this was the very thing she wanted to hear.

I offered him some sentences using affirmative language that celebrates the body. For example:

✳ 'I love the way you taste.'

✳ 'It turns me on when I'm eating you out/ going down on you/[insert your fave thing here].'

✳ 'You feel so good like that.'

✳ 'There's no rush – I've got all day/night for this.'

✳ 'Let's just do what feels good and remove the pressure to orgasm.'

✳ 'You don't have to worry about me – I'll let you know if I need to pause or take a break.'

✳ 'How can we make this feel even better for you?'

Learning this language outside of a sexual context was reassuring for them. He was able to fully enjoy giving, knowing it's not creepy, and she was able to relax into receiving.

YOUR BODY CAN TALK

Practising voicing your desires is an important skill, but it's just as important to understand nonverbal communication, like touch, eye contact, sounds, gestures, posture and even tone.

Here are some ways to reflect on your nonverbal communication methods:

✳ How can you show your partner you're listening?

✳ What do you notice/look for in your partner's body language to gauge how they're feeling?

✳ How can you use tone, gestures, looks and body language?

OPENING UP

Jake and Stuart had been together for five years. They'd been non-monogamous for most of their relationship, Jake booked in to see me, as he was finding it challenging to communicate openly with Stuart about his experiences with other partners. They'd stopped having sex together as it 'didn't feel right', and then started feeling awkward. Stuart struggled to trust Jake completely, fearing that important information was being withheld. In session with Jake, he practised voicing shame to me, naming it out loud and being witnessed, held and safe.

Jake was consistently at his learning edge. Although he wanted to run away and avoid the most uncomfortable conversations, he practised being honest to establish agreements that honoured each other's autonomy while maintaining a strong emotional connection. Stuart was vital in rewiring the fear of abandonment, as he proved he wasn't going to run away in the face of conflict or hard conversations.

We also brought a somatic approach to address Jake's internalised homophobia. After sex, he was often grossed out by the things he was doing, and this shame led him to hide it from the man he loved most.

His 'disgust' response made him want to crawl into a ball and hide himself. So I asked him to explore what it was like to allow his body to do just that. He crawled his body into a ball. In the ball he said he felt small, a little silly, but protected. He stayed there for a few minutes. I invited him, when he was ready, to slowly, and with breath, sequence his way out of this ball. Over about five minutes he moved from a tight ball into an open and strong standing position. This sounds so simple, and really it was. But afterwards, he reported feeling like his shame had been acknowledged; he didn't fight it, he held it company and then for the first time felt like he had choice around what he wanted to do with it.

He started to use this practice at home. When the disgust or shame response was triggered, he listened to his body and would intentionally move to a shape or posture that felt grounded and safe. It was from this place of safety and grounding that he was able to have more challenging conversations with Stuart.

Be specific

Most people love when their partner tells them what they want. A lot of the time we're just guessing what feels good for them, or inferring from the way they're moving, moaning or breathing. If you can communicate what you're into – the speed, rhythm, pace or type of touch you like – it can be a helpful mirror, encouraging your partner to share equally while creating an open, playful and non-judgemental space to explore.

Practice is essential

Things aren't going to change overnight – it's likely you'll need to practise communicating. And when you're learning together it shows that you're committed to working on it together. Doing the clunky, uncomfortable thing lets us practise being at our learning edge. Maybe start off by talking about what you like outside of a sexual context with something a little less vulnerable than a head between your legs. What about asking for a back rub or massage, or a touch or kiss on an erogenous zone.

Ask: Who is this for?

Many of us are familiar with feeling like we need to perform our pleasure for others – I often hear clients say, 'I don't want to make them feel like they're doing a bad job.' But all too often the person who is receiving is more focused on the giver's experience than their own pleasure at receiving. By asking 'Who is this for?' we're able to check in and notice whether we're enduring a position that's uncomfortable, putting up with touch that isn't really hitting the spot or going along with something because we're scared to offend. If they're a good sexual partner, they will want to touch you in the way you like, so give them all the information they need to do that.

Trust them

This goes for everyone. If someone says they like giving, or they love a certain sexual act, we need to learn to trust them. Many people love giving pleasure to their partner. It can turn them on, but it can also just feel really good knowing their partner feels good. So if someone says they want to do something, trust them.

PRAISE KINK

You've heard of dirty talk, but have you ever tried praise kink? They're not necessarily total opposites, but there is a distinct difference between the two.

✳ **Praise kink:** When a person finds compliments/words of affirmation/positive feedback arousing or pleasurable.

✳ **Dirty talk:** Any communication before/during/after sex that turns you on – can express needs, desires or turn-ons.

Praise kink	Dirty talk
✳ Affirmation-based ✳ Before, during or after sex	✳ Directive or responsive ✳ Before, during or after sex
'Good girl, boy, baby, mummy, daddy' 'I can't wait to show you off' 'I love it when you ...' 'You're so good at ...' 'I'm going to reward you for that' 'I want you so bad' 'You look/taste/feel so good'	'It turns me on when you ...' 'Touch/Bite/Hold me like this' 'Just wait until we get home' 'Tease me/Bend over/Right there' 'You've been bad and need to be punished' 'I want you' 'Fuck me'

How to talk about sex

I'm often asked *exactly* how to talk about sex. I know talking about it, trying something new or asking for what you want can feel tricky, so I developed this framework, showing how to structure a great sex conversation. Please note, this framework is designed for those who want to improve sex, but they're not sure where to start.

Context: When is a good time for you to talk? If you're talking about something you want to improve or change in your sexual relationship, I recommend not raising this right before, during or after sex – it can feel a little too vulnerable. Typically, people opt to have these conversations on a walk, at dinner or while sitting down with no distractions. But of course, this will be different for everyone.

The good stuff: This is really, *really* important. Tell your partner what you love (or really like) about your relationship, sex or each other. What is going well? Remind them of all the good things they do. These reminders are there to create a sense of ease. It's pretty common to only hear the bad stuff. Let's take the shit sandwich approach and start by naming all the good things – because I'm sure there are many.

Room for improvement: Notice the language here too. What we're really asking is, *What would make it better? What do you want to work on? What are you curious about and why do you want to do this new thing?* It'll also be about both sides taking responsibility. We can't come in and say, 'You never rub my clit the right way', especially if you've never given explicit and ongoing direction. Instead, this may sound like, 'I've noticed I'm not speaking up during sex. I want to be more explicit with the way you're rubbing my clit – I really like X and I don't like Y. Can I show you how?' This is the time for questions and information gathering.

Note: If they're doing something that is uncomfortable, painful or that you're really not into, you certainly don't need to frame this as an improvement. Be as explicit as you can: 'I don't like …' or 'Stop …' or 'I don't want to …'

Some more good stuff: Reiterate the good stuff, as a reminder of why you want to work on your relationship and to round off the shit sandwich (maybe we could rebrand this to the sex sandwich). This could be as simple as repeating what you've said, reminding them they're sexy, hot and great with their hands, and reassuring them – and yourself – that these check-ins and conversations are vital for a fulfilling relationship. Couples who speak about sex have better sex.

Allow for space: You don't need to come up with an answer straight away. Space can be an incredibly valuable tool, allowing each other to process. Just agree on a time when you'll continue the conversation, so you're not left feeling like you're in limbo.

Integrate: Consider this the aftercare of conversations. Thank each other for your openness, and finish by integrating with something physical, emotional, sensual, active or playful. Integration is anything over 30 seconds that allows your nervous systems to register the process you've been through. This may be a long cuddle, a kiss, affirming words or thanking each other. Build closeness and celebrate the fact that you both cared for each other and survived something that was challenging. Go you! Proud of you!

Now, these are the things I invite you to do with your body while talking about sex:

✳ **Breathe:** When we're stressed, we hold our breath, which induces anxiety. Try long, deep exhales.

✳ **Ease physical tension in your body:** Release tension in your jaw, pelvis and bum. Relax your shoulders away from your ears. You don't need to prepare for battle; you're just talking about sex to make it better for everyone. Physically, we can remind our bodies of this by releasing tension.

✳ **Ground:** This conversation does not mean you are unworthy, or a bad lover, or that you're not good enough. Remind yourself that talking about sex makes you a great lover, and working together makes for a really good sex life.

✳ **Physical touch:** For yourself or each other, this may be a hand on the knee, chest or stomach.

✳ **Look into each other's eyes:** This is simple, but so challenging. Couples will often divert attention, which instantly disconnects us and creates distance. You don't need to be staring into each other's soul the whole time. Look away, close your eyes, blink whenever you need to – just look back to each other when it feels okay.

✳ **Get up:** If you feel stuck or like you're talking in circles, get up, pause, shake or move your body. Go outside for a breath of fresh air and come back after a few moments. This is not leaving or fleeing the conversation, it's taking a few moments to reset and coming back when you feel more regulated.

It is so common to go into protection mode. It can feel scary initiating a conversation about sex; it can feel really scary when someone wants to talk about sex too. But even though it's scary, it's really important. Try to be proud of yourself for having a hard conversation.

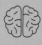

Speed relating

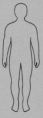

Early on in my career, I created a game called 'speed relating' as a way to lower the stakes and practise communication outside of a sexual context. I assign it to most couples. You'll need 30 to 60 mins and a timer. Take turns answering the questions below for one minute; no more, no less. When the timer goes, switch so your partner will answer the next question. You don't need to come up with an answer straight away. After you've heard the question, take a breath, stay with it and answer when you're ready.

* What does fulfilling sex mean to you?

* How do you like to be touched?

* What are your boundaries?

* What excites you?

* What turns you on?

* What turns you off?

* What touch do you like giving?

* What touch do you like receiving?

* How does it feel asking for what you want?

* What pressures have you felt in sex/ relationships?

* How sexually confident do you feel at the moment?

* What's your relationship like with sexual desire right now?

* Is there anything you know you never want to try during sex?

* What are you curious about when it comes to sex?

* What did you learn, notice and feel during this game?

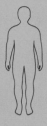

Questions to ask during sex

✳ What would make this even better?

✳ How would you like that?

✳ More of this?

✳ How's that?

✳ What are you noticing?

✳ Can you describe that in more detail?

✳ How's this pressure/vibration/speed/ rhythm/movement/touch?

✳ May I ...?

✳ Can you ...?

✳ Will you ...?

✳ How does that feel?

✳ Can we do something else?

✳ Less of that?

✳ Where do you want to be kissed?

✳ Is this exactly what you want?

✳ Are you still into this?

✳ Can you touch me here?

✳ Is this still exciting?

✳ Is this what you're looking for?

✳ Like this?

✳ Can you slow down?

✳ This is what I understood, but is this what you want?

✳ Can you ask for something else?

✳ What does your body want?

✳ Do you like that?

✳ Does that feel good?

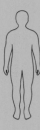

Statements during sex

※ I love it when you do that.

※ YES YES YES!

※ That's perfect.

※ Let's pause.

※ No thanks.

※ Stop.

※ More … Less … Up … Down … Deeper …
Slower … Harder … Softer …

※ That's enough.

※ No, *this* is what I want.

※ I want you to …

※ I want to …

※ Tell me what you want.

※ Fuck yes!

※ I won't touch you till you tell me.

※ Show me what you mean.

※ You turn me on when you do that.

※ I want to see you naked.

※ I'm so wet/hard when you do that.

※ Go back to what you were doing.

※ Faster, slower …

※ I need you to …

※ Tease me.

※ This is exactly what I want.

※ Tell me what to do.

※ Keep doing that.

※ Don't stop.

※ I've been so good/bad/naughty.

※ I love holding your dick/fingering you/
my fingers inside you …

※ You're going to make me cum.

※ You taste/feel so good!

IMPORTANT STUFF

✳ Sexual communication is a skill that often requires time and practice. It is also a tool that can help you work through most sex-related concerns.

✳ Start by talking about sex outside of a sexual context. This will lower the stakes and give you an opportunity to practise in a context that makes you feel less vulnerable.

✳ Take your time to learn about what it is that you want; this'll make it easier to ask for what you want during sex.

✳ A little reassurance can go a long way. Sexual communication skills can also be about reminding your partner that you love the way they look, taste and smell or that you will let them know if you need a break. This simple act of reassurance allows the person who's receiving to release into the moment.

✳ Sexual communication can also be really fucking hot. Talking about sex can feel like foreplay and can energise the sexual experience.

SAFER SEX

How do I discuss safer sex with
a one-night stand? How can we use
a condom without killing the mood?
How often do I need to get tested?

Safer sex is sexy, and it's an important part of your sexual
wellness. For many, practising safer sex helps them fully
relax into sexual experiences knowing they are prioritising
health and safety. I use the term *safer sex* rather than *safe
sex*, because no contraception or barrier method is 100 per
cent effective every time. But still, using some protection is
always safer than using none. Safer sex is sex that prevents
or limits the exchange of bodily fluids like semen, blood
and vaginal fluids between partners. This helps prevent
pregnancy and sexually transmitted infections, or STIs.

I often like to speak about sexual hygiene at the same time as safer sex, as they both fall under the umbrella of sexual wellness. Sexual hygiene is about making sure your body, toys, tools and the space where you're having sex are clean, to minimise the risk of transmitting bodily fluids and developing infections. It's also about creating a context for a really great sexual experience: making sure your sheets are clean, showering regularly and washing genitals with a body-safe soap, and cleaning and storing your toys in a proper toy bag to ensure they're ready to go each time. Simple hygiene and safer-sex practices ensure everyone leaves feeling great about the experience, rather than doubting or fearing what's to come.

As with all sexual experiences, there's a lot you can do to ensure you're having the safest sex possible. While there is nothing shameful or dirty about living with an STI – they are really common – it is important to be responsible for your sexual health and that of the people you are having sex with. This chapter includes a section addressing STI shame and stigma, including how best to approach conversations with partners.

HOW DO I HAVE SAFER SEX?

* **Condoms:** Use a barrier method like a condom every time you have vaginal, anal or oral sex or sex with toys to protect against STIs and (if there's a penis and vagina involved) unwanted pregnancies. Remember to use a fresh one each time, and store them in a cool, dry place away from sharp objects.

* **Dental dams and barrier methods:** A dental dam is a thin latex sheet that you can put on or in between genitals to act as a physical barrier, or other barrier methods (like cut-open condoms) can provide a protective barrier between you and your partner.

* **Lube:** Using lube every time you have sex will reduce the chances of the condom breaking, as well as reducing friction, discomfort and potential tears. Water-based and silicon-based lubes are recommended for use with condoms, but make sure you only use water-based lubes with toys because silicon lubes can degrade the material of silicon toys.

* **STI testing:** Regularly getting tested for STIs is an essential part of taking care of your sexual health. It's recommended to get tested for STIs once every 6 to 12 months, even if you're in a long-term relationship. You should test more often if you're having sex with multiple people or when you have sex with someone new. You can get tested at a GP, sexual health clinic, family planning clinic, community health centre or LGBTQIA+ sexual health clinic. Some STIs are asymptomatic, so you or others may transmit them without even realising it, which is why getting tested is important. A quick Google search will identify the sex-positive clinics in your area, and if you don't have one nearby, there are great online resources too.

* **Birth-control options:** If you're looking to prevent pregnancy, there are various birth-control methods available, from hormonal options like the pill, patch or implant, to non-hormonal choices like the copper IUD or condoms. Speak with your healthcare provider to find the best fit for you.

* **PrEP:** If you're at a higher risk of contracting HIV, pre-exposure prophylaxis (PrEP) might be worth discussing with your healthcare provider. This involves taking a daily medication to significantly reduce the risk of HIV transmission. PrEP is a pill that HIV-negative people can take to prevent acquiring HIV. Taking it before being exposed to HIV means there will be enough of the drug in your system to stop HIV if it gets into your body. It's safe, well tolerated, and approved by the TGA for use by people who are HIV negative. If you take it as prescribed, it can reduce the risk of HIV transmission by almost 100 per cent. Just be aware that it doesn't prevent other STIs or pregnancy.

BEFORE SEX

Safer sex is often a process and, as such, there are things we can do before, during and after sex. Before you get into bed with someone, you should already be thinking about how you prepare for sex. That means making sure you're getting tested regularly, considering your barrier method or birth-control options, and speaking with sexual partners about the contraception and protection you use. Doing this before you're about to have sex sets the tone and expectations.

If someone doesn't want to use your preferred method of contraception, you have a few options. You could ask them how they like to practise safer sex, and then decide if that suits you too. You could find something that works for everyone involved. And of course, it may be non-negotiable for you. It's perfectly reasonable to decide you don't want to have sex with someone if they're not open to your safer-sex practice of choice. I know it can feel challenging to assert a boundary. This is what it could sound like:

Comment: 'Sex doesn't feel good with a condom on.'

Response: 'Sex doesn't feel good when I'm worried about STIs or unwanted pregnancy.'

Comment: 'Condoms don't fit me.'

Response: 'I've seen videos where people put their whole arm and leg in a condom. It'll fit you.'

Comment: 'I don't want to have sex with protection.'

Response: 'Then I don't want to have sex with you.'

DURING SEX

You don't really need to think about the pill, Implanon and PrEP during sex, but you do need to think about barrier methods, as they can rip or tear. If this happens, and bodily fluid is outside of the barrier method, it can still get into your mouth, anus or vagina. So make sure you're checking between sex positions. You can also pause and readjust at any time to make sure it's comfy for you. If you're in a group sex dynamic, or you're using toys with others, change the condom with each new partner. It's also really important to change the condom during anal sex, be it a penis, toy or fingers, before moving it to any other body part.

Sex can get messy, and for many, it's the mess of it all that's a turn on. If unwanted bodily fluids get into your mouth, eye, vagina or anus, you can rinse that area with water to flush it away, but it's important to remember this does not reduce the chance of pregnancy or STIs.

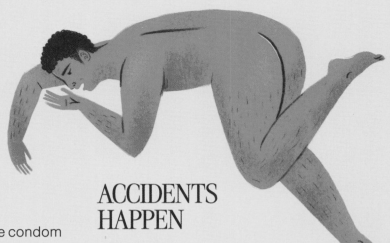

AFTER SEX

Immediately after sex, remove the condom or dental dam you've been using and throw it away. Don't re-use it – if you want to go again, put on a fresh condom. Make sure you clean your toys and accessories with a toy cleaner and store them in a place that's free from dust and bacteria. It's also highly recommended that you pee after sex to minimise the chances of a urinary tract infection, or UTI.

For people with vulvas, the urethra is very close the vagina, and for people with penises, the urethra is the same tube they ejaculate from, so it's really easy to transfer bacteria from the genitals to the urethra. If it stays there, it can cause a UTI.

UTIs can feel uncomfortable and painful, and can also lead to pretty serious health problems if left untreated. If you're experiencing prolonged discomfort or pain after sex, it's always best to see your GP.

ACCIDENTS HAPPEN

Sometimes sex just doesn't go according to plan. Condoms can break, dental dams can move out of place, sometimes you forget to take the pill. You're human. But you do have a responsibility to care for the people you have sex with. Here's what to do if something goes wrong:

1. **Talk about it.** Tell them what happened. 'It looks like the condom has ripped; let's stop for a moment,' or 'I realised the other night that I had forgotten to take my pill the weekend we had sex.'

2. **Discuss next steps together.** As sex was something you did together, often it can be kind to problem-solve together. You might need to get emergency contraception or an STI test.

3. **Keep them in the loop.** If your STI test returns a positive result, tell the person you had sex with, as well as any other recent sexual partners. A phone call or in-person conversation is often best, even though I know it can feel nerve-racking.

HOW TO TALK ABOUT STIs

With so much misinformation and stigma surrounding STIs, it can feel pretty daunting to speak about them. But STIs are statistically very common. It's estimated that around one in six people will get an STI in their lifetime. I want to make this very, very clear: an STI doesn't say anything about who you are as a person. You are not dirty or unworthy of love and mind-blowing sex. You deserve a loving relationship and really good sex just as much as everyone else. And while it may feel hard to talk about, stats consistently prove that open conversations around sexual health actively lessen the risk of STI transmission. Research also shows us that people who disclose their STI to their partners have more positive feelings towards their sexual self-esteem than those who don't disclose. Speaking openly about STIs removes the shame and stigma, and means it's not something you need to navigate on your own. Unfortunately, none of us were taught how to have these conversations.

I know it's easier said than done, but it's important. And we're practising being vulnerable, right?! How you approach it will be entirely up to you. Often a little prep goes a long way, so speak with sexual partners in a way that feels safe and comfy for you. Here are a couple of shame-free ways you can approach telling a potential fling about your STI.

Know the facts

We should really be taught this stuff at school, but because we're not, it's important to do your own research, especially if you have an STI or you're sleeping with someone who has one. It can be overwhelming enough meeting someone new; starting a discussion around STIs and sexual health can be enough to make you want to run away. But by speaking with a sex-positive health practitioner, doing your research and knowing all the important information, you're doing the groundwork for a healthy sexual relationship. If you don't know how to manage and practise safer sex with an STI, you really can't expect the people you're having sex with to know either.

As well as doing your STI research, it may be useful to research different community groups, be it a private online group, a regular meet-up or a group therapy situation organised by a trusted professional.

There are lots of options if you're not able or willing to attend in person, so look into what may be useful for you or ask your GP if they have any recommendations. Having access to conversations with people with a similar lived experience can be a useful resource for gathering positive and shame-free information. It can also reassure you that you too can have a healthy and fulfilling sex life.

Try not to take a bad reaction to heart

The way they respond is giving you information about them, not about you. There's no way to know how someone will respond. They may have their own shame and stigma about STIs, because let's face it, growing up, who was taught anything useful about how to manage them?

But I have faith in humanity. There are so, so many mature, kind and informed people who will still respect and value you, and will be keen to discuss how you can have really good sex together. If they respond in a way that is hurtful or judgemental, let them know how their reaction is affecting you, and then present them with the correct information to help them understand. That said, if their reaction is an indication that they're not the kind of person you want to have sex with, you may not want to spend time educating them.

So it may go really well, or it may be subpar. Once you've had the conversation, give yourself a pat on the back or shout yourself a treat, because, well done. You're an upstanding sexual citizen. You've done your bit to break down the stigma, shame and misinformation around STIs, which reduces the risk of transmission. Importantly, I want to remind you that you can and will have a really fulfilling, fun and sexy life. And if at times you can't include your genitals, get creative (the best lovers do).

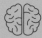

How to discuss safer sex

The hook-up

✳ 'I know we've just met, but seeing as we've been hooking up, can I ask you a question about safer-sex practices?'

✳ 'I'm really attracted to you and want to ask you something …'

✳ 'I'm really into this, and you. I want to be safe, and I like to use [insert your preferred safer-sex practice]'

✳ 'Before we go any further, how do you want to be safe together?'

Someone you're dating

✳ 'I'm really into this and want to do more, but wanted to check in with you first. Would you like to have sex? If that's something you're into, I'd love for both of us to get screened for STIs.'

✳ 'Do you want to go back to mine? I've got condoms/dental dams, lube and a whole box of toys so just bring yourself.'

✳ 'Safer sex really turns me on. How do you want to keep it safe?'

Friends with benefits

✳ 'I really enjoyed going down on you last weekend. As we've agreed this is a casual thing, I'd like to start playing with protection. I want to use X. What do you want to use?'

✳ 'Thinking about you in my bed and how hot it was when you reached for the condoms.'

✳ 'Do you know what would make this even better? Protection.'

Long-term partner

✳ 'I know we've been doing it the same way for a while, but it's really important for me to be safe when it comes to sex. Can we start using these [insert safer-sex practice of choice]?'

✳ 'I love having sex with you. I have noticed we're not exactly being safe, though; let's start doing that again.'

✳ 'Nothing turns me on more than trying something new. Let's use protection.'

IMPORTANT STUFF

✳ Safer sex is sexy, and knowing you're doing everything you can to take care of your health and that of others can bring enormous peace of mind.

✳ STIs are statistically really common. You can still have great sex and relationships while living with an STI.

✳ Having an STI doesn't say anything about who you are as a person; you are not dirty or unworthy of love and mind-blowing sex.

✳ You can and will have a really fulfilling, fun and sexy life.

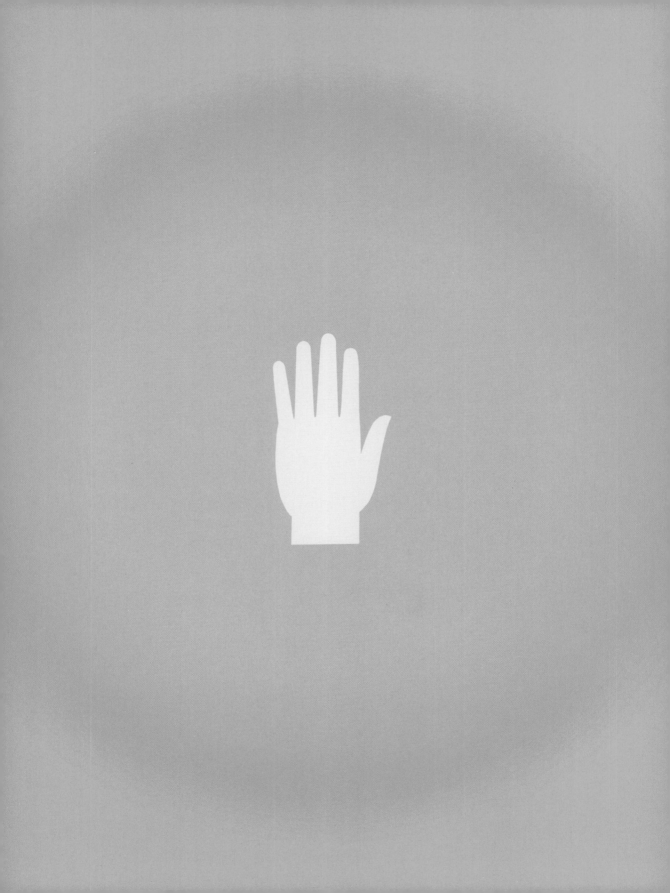

FOREPLAY AND AFTERCARE

Why does it take me so long to climax? How can I make the whole experience of sex feel better? What can I do if I feel low after sex? In this chapter we're looking at how to nail the process of sex, how understanding your unique arousal pattern can make everything feel better, how to improve foreplay and why every single one of us needs more aftercare.

I have issues with the way we foreplay. My first concern is that we conflate outercourse and foreplay – they're not the same thing. Foreplay is often considered to be all the stuff we do before penetrative sex: dry humping, touching, oral, hand stuff. But all these things *are* sex. Sure, they may be classified as outercourse, but defining sex as penetration alone is heteronormative, exclusive and, quite frankly, boring.

My second issue is in how we currently foreplay. Foreplay is so much more than just 30 seconds of fingering that leads to fast penetration. Foreplay actually serves an essential purpose in great sex, as it connects our minds and our bodies. It's powerful and important. I spend a lot of my time in session with couples working to integrate more foreplay into their lives as a tool for better sex.

I think there are ways we can use or redefine the concept of foreplay. My supervisor Deej Juventin puts it this way: 'Foreplay is getting our nervous systems in sync.' Foreplay can be moments of attunement, communication, co-regulating your nervous systems, establishing a shared sense of desire, creating context for desire, sending a flirty text. As Esther Perel famously states, foreplay starts at the end of the previous orgasm. Foreplay is all about what you do to build arousal and create the context for desire.

WHY FOREPLAY?

Foreplay builds arousal in our bodies, which makes touch feel better. Kissing triggers the release of feelgood neurochemicals, which can lower our inhibitions, reduce the stress hormone cortisol and support us in feeling more connected. It helps us attune with others; it's fun, brings sex front of mind and keeps sex exciting and playful. I could go on, but I'm guessing you get it. It's really useful to understand how arousal and foreplay work together. We'll look at understanding arousal later in this chapter.

And if your partner isn't interested? Give them this book. Seriously. They need to do some work to learn how to be a good lover. All sexual partners should be interested in foreplay, it's a really important part of great sex. You can't do this on your own.

EMOTIONAL INTIMACY VS SEXUAL INTIMACY

I was once working with a young queer couple who had moved in together after two weeks of dating. At the start of their relationship, sex was really fun, regular and impassioned. But after living together for a while, they noticed sex had dropped off their radar completely. Their relationship was still intimate, they kissed and cuddled and expressed love constantly, but because there was so much emotional intimacy, they noticed there was no drive for sex. And while emotional intimacy is important in long-term love, they had to work to create more sexual intimacy as a drive for sexual experiences.

It can be jarring when we feel intimately connected and close to someone but we don't want to have sex with them. It's hard to initiate sexual intimacy with someone after discussing the overdue energy bill while they do a shit. Sexual intimacy is not about being naked – in fact, sometimes it can feel more intense with clothes on as they act as a barrier. It's also useful for those who want to feel sexually close to their partner but aren't in the space for anything more intense or penetrative. And I know I've referenced a long-term relationship here, but this goes for everyone. Building sexual intimacy during a one-night stand can make it far more memorable.

HOW TO BUILD SEXUAL INTIMACY

Sexual intimacy is a kind of intimacy or closeness that relates to eroticism, pleasure and desire. It's something I talk a lot about in session with couples who are in love (think kisses, cuddles, emotional intimacy, support – all the good stuff)

but have stopped having sex. It can bridge the gap between all those sensitive, connected things and wanting to fuck someone on date night.

It's not about being naked. Practising sexual intimacy is great for people who want to put desire back on the map and build arousal within a relationship. It's also useful for those who want to feel close to their partner but aren't in the space for anything more intense or penetrative. Sexual intimacy can be built through the following simple acts of erotic awareness.

Make out more

At the start of a relationship, couples may spend hours just kissing with tongue, lost in each other's mouths. Many of my clients say they miss this, and sometimes they just want to make out on the couch without the need to have sex afterwards. Swap the standard peck for tongue and remove the pressure for it to go anywhere else.

Pro tip: Set a timer for a couple of minutes and keep kissing for the duration, pausing or checking in when the timer goes off.

Dry humping

Dry humping is where you grind against your partner, with clothes on, to increase sensation and arousal. It can feel really exciting to have a physical barrier between you and avoids the intensity or sensitivity of genitals touching. Experiment with moving your hips and using motions like gyrating, grinding or thrusting.

Pro tip: Explore holding non-genital erogenous zones with sensual touch – the hips, the back of the neck, chest, face, stomach and inner thighs are all great places to start.

Have a shower together

Sounds simple enough – and that's because it is. Showering together can be a really intimate act. Not just because you're saving the planet and reducing your water bill (seriously), but because you're wet and touching and enjoying each other's bodies without the expectation of sex.

Pro tip: Try washing each other's hair or body.

Sexual compliments (outside of sex)

That means complimenting your partner – on their body, their mind, what you love about them, how they make you feel – without any intention or expectation of sex. This may sound like:

✳ 'The way you talk turns me on.'

✳ 'You looked so sexy this morning.'

✳ 'I know I should be working, but I can't stop thinking about you.'

✳ 'You're perfect to me, I love every inch of your body.'

✳ 'You're so hot.'

✳ 'It really turns me on when you do that.'

✳ 'I love your [favourite body part].'

Sexual intimacy is the precursor to great sexual experiences, and not nearly enough people are engaging with it. This is foreplay in its finest form, and it's a non-negotiable when it comes to good sex.

FOREPLAY: DOs AND DON'Ts

Do:

✳ Redefine: Foreplay is so much more than the moments before sex, or something you do to arrive at an end goal. Foreplay can be the way you touch or kiss with your partner throughout the day, the engaging conversation shared over dinner, a knowing glance, talking about what you're into. It can be sharing a song, a steamy text, a hand on the lower back. Redefine foreplay together.

✳ Extend it: Generally, everyone speeds through foreplay. The more build-up and anticipation, the more intense it'll feel.

✳ Go beyond genitals: Arouse the whole body before going anywhere near their genitals, experiment with a variety of touch: teasing, holding, awakening sensation, kissing, etc.

✳ Experiment: Trying new things is an erotic energiser. Try incorporating toys, different kinds of touch or temperature into the mix.

✳ Come prepared: Have your barrier methods, tools and lube close by so you're ready.

✳ Stay present: I know this is easier said than done, but when you find yourself drifting away from the moment (or thinking about the dirty dishes in the sink), try incorporating some grounding or mindfulness techniques such as body awareness, focusing on touch, pausing to connect back in or changing the way you're moving.

Don't:

✳ Rush it: Take your time building arousal, excitement and connection.

✳ Assume: Keep a steady stream of communication throughout, instead of assuming how people want to be touched. Ask: 'How do you want to be kissed/touched?' 'What would make this better?' 'What turns you on?'

✳ Pressure: Remove pressure from yourself or your partner to respond in a certain way. Every sexual experience is different, and it's likely your body will respond in different or surprising ways each time you have sex.

✳ Perform: Foreplay is not a performance, it's a co-created experience. If their touch isn't hitting the spot, try being descriptive in what would work for you – a change in pace, technique, rhythm or pressure can make all the difference.

AFTERCARE

So often after sex, we might roll off our partner, check our phone, get up and move on with our day. Aftercare is the essential moment before that happens. It doesn't have to mean lovingly gazing into their eyes talking about how obsessed you are – this may not be fitting for, say, a one-night stand – but it is an important moment of integration that allows you to connect and check in afterwards. It reminds us that we're human beings who shared something.

The concept and practice of aftercare was introduced by BDSM folk (we can learn a lot about great sex from our kinky friends), and it has since been used outside of these communities. At its core, aftercare ensures everyone feels cared for after sex – moments that can feel vulnerable, shameful or intense for many. Even when sex has been consensual and we've willingly taken part, we may experience shame or guilt. This can be eased through co-regulation, communication and care.

Some people are more prone to feeling low, sad or depressed after sex – we call this postcoital dysphoria, also known as post-sex blues. When you're having sex, your body is flooded with feelgood neurochemicals like serotonin, dopamine and oxytocin, which means after sex or orgasm, you're basically coming off a high. This can explain the drop in feeling good. Aftercare is a tool for creating safety and connection to ease this low as the chemicals dissipate.

Aftercare also promotes sexual satisfaction in relationships, as it helps us maintain intimacy to ensure our emotional needs are met, and bridges the gap between our sexual experiences and our everyday lives. We're the same person, and aftercare reminds us of this. It can help to think about foreplay as getting our minds and bodies in sync, and aftercare as a process of re-regulating. There are no rules on how to practise this; it's more important to figure out what you need most in that moment. Things you may want to try could include:

✳ cuddling while having a chat about what felt good

✳ giving each other arm tickles or a massage

✳ getting your partner a towel

✳ looking in each other's eyes

✳ making a meal together

✳ having a nap in each other's arms.

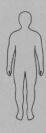

Dry humping

Dry humping is a non-penetrative sexual activity where you grind against another person or object to build arousal and even orgasm. In the era of forgotten foreplay, I want to celebrate dry humping as a pleasure essential – a kind of outercourse that can increase sensation (in a way that feels good enough to be the main course).

I recommend it for these reasons:

✳ It builds tension and anticipation. A barrier between genitals (i.e. your clothes) can feel more pleasurable than direct genital contact, which for some can be too intense. It can also build tension and anticipation, feel naughty/intimate/intense while also valuing outercourse as feeling as good, if not better than intercourse.

✳ It encourages movement. Sex can become quite rigid. Many people hold a lot of tension in their legs, pelvic floor and glutes, and while a tension orgasm can feel good, often adding movements like gyrating and grinding can help us build arousal in our genitals, release into pleasure and actively position our bodies so we get direct stimulation to the most sensitive areas.

✳ It slows us down. We can be quick to rush into sex. Dry humping slows us down, allows for connection and acts as foreplay, outercourse, intensifying sensation and arousal.

✳ It lets us make out with our clothes on. We may not always feel like naked, penetrative sex, but a good sesh of dry humping can tick all the boxes. It can also remind us of the enthusiasm of a new relationship, where bodies feel exciting, novel and electric. Full steam ahead!

Positions and technique

✳ **Missionary:** Lying down with one partner on top of the other allows for full-body contact and directly stimulates the genitals.

✳ **The leg-grind:** One partner lies or sits down and the other straddles their leg, knee or hip to ride, grind and stroke.

✳ **Straddle:** One partner lies on their back and the other sits on top, grinding back and forward, stimulating both their genitals and their partner's.

✳ **The rock 'n' roll:** This is a masturbation and humping must-have, courtesy of the pioneering sex educator Betty Dodson. The rock 'n' roll technique involves rocking the pelvis forward while squeezing the pelvic floor muscle, then rocking back and relaxing. You may wish to sync this with your breath – breathe in while you rock forward and squeeze, exhale as you rock back and release.

Quick tips

✳ **Wear comfortable clothes:** Choose materials that are comfortable to grind on.

✳ **Be creative:** Dry humping isn't just about the genitals. Touch, hold, bring them closer or keep them at a distance.

✳ **Experiment with slowly removing clothing:** Be mindful of how sensation changes as you add/remove pieces of clothing.

✳ **Switch it up:** Explore different rhythms, pressure and positions.

✳ **Increase the vibe:** Add vibrators, toys, sensory items, lube, blindfolds, etc. to increase sensation.

✳ **Do it naked:** Without clothes it's more like 'wet' humping. Add enough lube, so your genitals can glide and slide with ease.

IMPORTANT STUFF

✳ For many, foreplay is an essential element of great sex. It allows everyone involved to build arousal in their bodies.

✳ People aren't getting enough foreplay – it should be way more than just 30 seconds of kissing before you launch into hard and fast penetration.

✳ Foreplay looks different for everyone; it can involve intellectual, emotional and physical stimulation to build arousal.

✳ In longer term relationships, foreplay often falls off the priority list and as a result people desire sex less. They need time to get into their bodies and to connect with their partner. Most people aren't doing enough of this.

✳ Foreplay and outercourse are not the same thing.

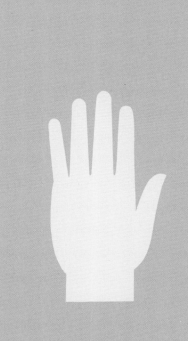

DESIRE

Why don't we do it anymore? What's up with my sex drive? How do we navigate mismatched libidos? Is there something wrong with me? Or you? Or us? Every person who has sex will ask questions like this. We've all been there – and if you haven't yet, it's likely you will.

Struggling with desire is one of the most common reasons couples seek professional support. The good news is, there are some really practical things you can do to reframe desire and help you want to *do it* more. We have a very linear understanding of desire; we've been taught to believe that when you like or love someone, you just want to bang each other at any given moment and you both want it at exactly the same time – but it doesn't necessarily work like this. Imagine if we applied this same thinking to dinner. Do you always want the exact same meal, in the same way, at the exact same time as your partner? No, of course you don't.

It is so predictably and *statistically* normal to go through periods where you're not having sex as often as you'd like. Relationships are complex and ever-evolving, and so is our desire for sex. It's common for couples to find themselves in this predicament; they deeply love and care for one another, but no longer feel the insatiable desire to inhale each other. *Is it normal that we're not having sex? Can love and low sexual desire coexist harmoniously?* Yes, it is – and yes, they can. Here are a few things to keep in mind.

WHAT IS DESIRE?

Sexual desire is a longing, wanting or motivation for sex. It can feel all-consuming. It's important to clarify language here. Desire is not a drive; sex is not a drive. Emily Nagoski, author of *Come as You Are*, states: 'A drive is a biological mechanism whose job is to keep the organism at a healthy baseline – not too warm, not too cold, not too hungry, not too full.' Basically, you will die if you don't drink water, eat food, sleep or breathe. But you won't die if you don't have sex. It's inaccurate and dangerous to refer to desire as a drive. Nagoski is a pioneer who's completed extensive research and

education on desire. She has changed the way we understand and speak about desire. I'll refer to her work often in this chapter, but for a more in-depth dive into desire, read *Come as You Are*.

There are two different ways of experiencing desire:

✳ **Spontaneous desire**: A spontaneous urge for sex that seemingly comes out of nowhere; it arises spontaneously and without external stimulation. My clients often say it feels like a sudden urge or craving that emerges with little or no stimulus. We see this a lot in porn and in movies, and often experience it at the start of a relationship. It could be prompted by a quick thought or something mental, followed by rapid physiological arousal: 'I just thought about having sex ... and now I'm turned on.' Some people experience spontaneous desire fairly frequently, while others may experience it less often, or not at all.

✳ **Responsive desire**: A type of sexual desire that emerges in response to external or internal cues. Rather than feeling an innate urge, those who are responsive may experience desire after engaging in sexual stimuli, like receiving neck kisses for a few minutes, feeling emotionally connected to their partner, thinking about something erotic or even watching a sex scene. You respond to certain stimuli and then you think, 'Oh, yes, sex, this is a great idea!' Responsive desire occurs when someone may not actively seek out a sexual encounter, but they're into it when presented with the right context and stimuli. It is important to note that responsive desire is just as valid and common as spontaneous desire, but may be less frequently discussed or understood. This challenges the notion that sexual desire should always be spontaneous. In this case, the mental desire often comes after the physical response.

Both types of desire are sexy, healthy and normal. I notice in session that working through these different types of desire can help my clients navigate and communicate their desires within relationships. However, there's an expectation that we should all be spontaneous in our desire, when in reality, the majority of us are responsive.

Desire exists on a spectrum, and we all experience it differently. So rather than neatly fitting into a category or a type, we can map out how we relate to sex and desire based on the spectrum shown below. Where would you place your desire style?

Spontaneous ———————————————————————— Responsive

For others, it may feel a bit more like this:

Spontaneous

Responsive

Desire is not necessarily one or the other. Sometimes you're responsive, sometimes you're spontaneous. When I explain this to my clients it's like they have a lightbulb moment. They've been waiting for desire to smack them in the face, without recognising that they may need to actively create the context for themselves and their partner.

This distinction is important. When I work through it in session, my clients share statements like these:

✳ 'I'm so relieved to understand that I'm responsive – I thought I was broken, but maybe I'm just not receiving or actively engaging in the stimulus I need.'

✳ 'I thought I was too much because I was desiring sex more than my partner. I thought there was something wrong with me.'

✳ 'We thought that because we desired sex differently, our bodies were trying to tell us something. We thought we weren't compatible.'

TWO COMMON CONCERNS

Low libido

This is all relative, and unfortunately how we understand low and high desire is based on how we compare ourselves to others. I'll often hear people say, 'I'm usually the one with higher desire, but now I'm not', or 'I just can't keep up with them'. Often my clients will report having 'low libido', but more often than not, when we work through the science behind desire, they'll realise they're actually more responsive in their desire, and they're not receiving the stimulus they need. They're not actively creating a context for desire, and as a result, they desire sex very rarely.

As no two people are the same, it's important to learn about your normal, and discover what we call a desire baseline. For some, normal is desiring sex every day. For others it's a few times a week, a few times a month, or every few months. We cannot, and should not, compare our desire and our relationships to other people's – we will all have different ideas about what a healthy and fulfilling sex life means. It's also really common for this to change. Sometimes one person desires sex more, and then this shifts.

153

Desire discrepancy

This is often referred to as 'mismatched libido', but I prefer to use the term desire discrepancy because 'mismatch' is such a loaded term. You are not 'mismatched' because you desire sex at different times or with differing frequency. Desire is a motivational system, a wanting for something. You're not broken if you want sex less than your partner; perhaps you experience desire differently.

We all have things that turn us off and on. When working with this, we need to start with a plan to create a context where desire can thrive. We also need to look at your sexual excitation system (accelerators) and sexual inhibition system (brakes), as discussed in Chapter 4, and examine what you and your partner can do to bring more accelerators and limit some of the brakes. Share your lists of brakes and accelerators with each other so you can identify areas where you overlap and how you can work together. After all, some people have more barriers to pleasure than others.

LEARNING ABOUT WHAT TURNS YOU ON AND OFF

According to Nagoski, sexual desire is a multifaceted and dynamic phenomenon influenced by a wide range of factors, both internal and external. These factors interact in complex ways, making it essential to recognise that changes in sexual desire are a normal part of the human experience. Nagoski emphasises that sexual desire is not a simple on–off switch, but rather a complex interplay of various components, including sexual arousal, emotional connection, stress levels, relationship dynamics and personal experiences. So we can't just sit around and wait for our desire to reappear – we have to start with some self-enquiry.

Remember Nagoski's dual-control model (which we discussed in Chapter 4)? Sexual desire has two components: sexual excitation (what turns us on) and sexual inhibition (what turns us off). While sexual excitation can be triggered by factors like arousal and attraction, sexual inhibition is influenced by external stressors, emotional states and relationship dynamics. An increase in inhibition can lead to a decrease in sexual desire.

For example, when you first start dating, you're engaging in exciting and thrilling activities like getting ready for a date or sending flirty messages throughout the day. Dating can feel uncertain, exciting and risky. We spend a lot of time thinking about this other person and waiting for the moment we will see or touch them next, which often energises our experiences. And while there's so much beauty in long-term relationships and long-term love, when couples move into more mundane patterns of relating – paying bills together, cleaning the house, arguing about whose turn it is to cook – it may no longer feel 'thrilling' to connect.

Understanding your dual-control model can help you and your partner understand each other's unique interplay between sexual excitation and inhibition, and look at ways to manage or remove some of the brakes and bring in more accelerators. Next, we need to create an ideal context for sex.

CONTEXT IS EVERYTHING

This seems so simple, and it's often trivialised and simplified in sealed section-esque columns: 'light a candle, clean your room, have a shower, massage each other'. Many people think about desire like a magic trick – you love someone and all of a sudden it should just appear, right? If only. The context in which sexual desire arises is crucial. External factors like stress, fatigue or relationship conflicts can contribute to the activation of sexual inhibition. So even if you love your partner deeply, you may experience a decrease in sexual desire due to the turn-offs at play. These might include a long to-do list, the mental load, harsh lighting, or having housemates, family members or kids close by. All these things can feel like a wet blanket for your desire.

Create the context for desire

Do things (big or small) that allow you to feel more sensual. For best results, try to make it a regular or daily practice. I know that seeing the word 'daily' can feel daunting, but here I'm really talking about sensual moments: kiss your partner with tongue, listen to erotica on your way home from work, create a sensual space for yourself or your partner, do things that are exciting and new, talk about sex more, and try taking the goal of 'orgasm' out of sex and focusing on intimacy and pleasure instead.

155

I WANT TO WANT IT

I was working with a couple in their mid-thirties. She'd just had a baby and was back working full-time. For over a decade, she'd pushed through painful sex due to vaginismus and endo. When I asked her why she was in session, she said to me, 'I want to want it.' This response is incredibly common. It recognises that right now sex is so far down the priority list, or so far beyond something that feels exciting, but they feel it's important for them, their partner and their relationship.

My client spoke about a time when she was a sexual person, when it felt fun and freeing. She felt like she'd lost herself. But as I was listening to what was going on in her life – new baby, working full-time, fear of painful sex – it made a lot of sense to me that she wasn't desiring sex. Sex had become this thing that could be uncomfortable, stressful, awkward and may even inflict unwanted pain. For her, there was no motivation for sex, but there was a motivation to shut it down and protect herself.

It's worth noting that her husband was supportive, kind, loving and patient. He was in no way pushing her to do something she didn't want to do, but he also saw value in working on their sexual relationship. In their first session we started by creating context for the motivation for sex. With motivation comes reward, which reinforces the cycle of wanting more. We needed to address how she could want it more.

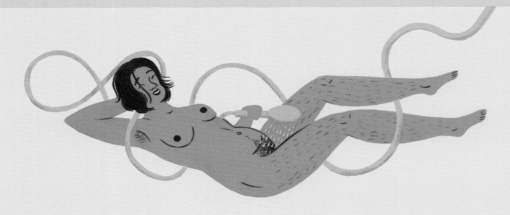

WORKING TOGETHER WITH A PARTNER

Often it's the person with self-diagnosed 'low desire' who books in the session with me. We've been socialised to think that the person who has a 'high drive' for sex is normal and the person with a lower desire for sex is 'biologically abnormal', as one cis heterosexual male client once referred to his partner. This is reductive and doesn't take into consideration a suite of factors important for a healthy and fulfilling sex life. Desire discrepancy is a relational concern. Both people will have different responsibilities to create a context for desire, so more often than not, I want them both in the room.

TAKE SEX OFF THE CARDS

Whenever a couple comes to see me about desire, I assign them the experiment of taking sex off the cards between our sessions. This may sound counterintuitive – after all, they're often seeing me because they want to have more sex – but I do this for a few reasons. Often, the person with lower desire for sex is so cautious of giving their partner the 'wrong idea' that they start to withdraw any kind of sensual or sexual

intimacy. They stop kissing their partner, they stop telling them they look sexy. They stop touching them. They fear that if they do any of these things, that may suggest that they want to have sex, and then they'll have to go through the whole process of saying no, feeling guilty and letting their partner down. However, this means they also miss out on doing many of the things that they love with their partner, like kissing, giving them compliments and feeling sexy. Similarly, their partner misses out on receiving these things, and on feeling wanted and feeling connected.

As a result, the couple limits the opportunity to create a context for desire together. They're not touching or kissing, talking about sex or thinking about sex. They exist in this space that is completely void of any sensual or sexual stimulus. To address this, we need to take the pressure off. We want to remove the fear of guilt, the fear of letting their partner down, and we want to explore different ways to create a context for desire. The easiest way to do this is to take penetrative sex off the cards for an agreed amount of time. But they are invited to experiment with daily moments of sensual pleasure. They're not having sex as they know it, but they are being sexual.

157

Instead, they come back to focusing on how they want to be touched or kissed, telling their partner what they love about them, and what they find sexy or attractive about them. Basically, we want to create a safe environment that is free from pressure and free from an end goal. In my experience, couples find that after doing this experiment, they are more sexually fulfilled, feel more connected and, importantly, feel a sense of hope that things can get better.

REDEFINE SEX

How can you invite intimate or pleasurable moments into your relationship beyond 'naked bodies penetrating each other'? A passionate kiss, naked massage, oral sex, dry humping ... these can all be fulfilling sexual experiences. Start having 'sex' that is exciting and fulfilling, and that focuses on the quality of the experience rather than the quantity or goal.

I have found that it is the couples who prioritise sex who have the most consistently fulfilling sex lives. They value it, they agree it's important for their relationship, they recognise that it may not always be front of mind, and it may change over time, but they commit to doing

things for themselves and their partner to make it a priority. They will stay in bed on a Saturday morning rather than go to the gym, they will leave the washing pile for an extra hour, they will set a date night and have sex before they go out because they know they'll be too tired and full by 10 pm. They share at-home tasks equally because they know that the mental load is real and heavy, particularly for cis women in heterosexual relationships, and they know it's hard to prioritise sex when you're stressed and thinking about everyone else. They recognise the reward cycle and try to make sex about fun, pleasure and feeling good, rather than about performance and pressure.

But this doesn't just have to be about prioritising getting naked and doing penetrative sex. Couples who engage in frequent and playful sexual moments are the most sexually fulfilled long term; they are more sexually satisfied than couples who have frequent and unfulfilling penetrative sex.

SEEKING SUPPORT

It can be useful to work through what's affecting your desire – relational changes, stress, bodies changing, moving into new stages of life, meeting someone else ... Really, there's so much here. I can't give you a blueprint approach without really knowing you – but a professional can.

If professional support isn't right for you right now, maybe start with some solo enquiry in the form of journalling, feeling into it or talking it through with a trusted person. Ask yourself: *How do I experience desire? What's changed in my relationship? What turns me on? What turns me off? When am I (or when was I) most attracted to them? When do I feel most attractive?*

REBUILDING FROM SCRATCH

Amira and Kate, a young queer couple, had been together for two years when they booked to see me. At the start of their relationship, they couldn't keep their hands off each other. Initially, they were playful, curious and focused on exploration and pleasure, but when Amira started speaking openly about her past sexual experiences, Kate began to feel inadequate. For the first time, sex became stressful. Kate felt like she couldn't live up to Amira's past relationships or her current needs. These concerns led to Kate avoiding sex, perpetuating a cycle of decreased sexual activity and increased anxiety.

This avoidance led Amira to think Kate was falling out of love with her, and that she didn't find her attractive. Amira also stopped initiating because she didn't feel wanted. She didn't think she'd been oversharing; she viewed it as an attempt to talk about the things she liked, in order to open up more dialogue about her wants, needs and desires during sex. This was her way of communicating her longing for Kate and the sexual intimacy they once shared, her yearning for the closeness and physical connection.

They were both feeling frustrated and let down, and they wanted more. Their desire for more sexual experiences was rooted in a need for emotional and physical connection.

In our sessions together, we focused on these areas:

✳ **Building and maintaining their communication and emotional connection:** They weren't speaking about sex before our sessions; it was too scary and always ended in a fight. We practised active listening, self-regulation while holding space, the art of sharing information while intending to do no harm, and being aware of the boundaries they set around what was too much information.

✳ **Exploring desire discrepancy:** We worked through many of the practices in this chapter, educating them about desire discrepancy and desire existing on a spectrum, and exploring how they could work together to create the context for desire.

✳ **Rebuilding sexual intimacy:** They took sex off the cards for a month and developed sexual intimacy away from sexual performance through acts such as showering each other's bodies, flirting with each other, kissing and grinding on the couch.

✳ **Learning together:** An exciting element for them was exploring new sexual experiences that neither of them were an 'expert' in, which levelled the playing field. They started to bring more creativity and play back to sex and removed the loaded titles of 'experienced' and 'less experienced'.

Finding your desire baseline

The baseline for 'normal' desire is different for everyone, and it's not useful to compare how often we want sex to how often others do. But it is useful to understand your desire baseline. This can help you track changes, be realistic and work towards a sex life that is fulfilling for you, rather than setting a goal based on an arbitrary quota you think you need to meet to maintain a good relationship. To understand yours, reflect on the following questions.

✳ What is your 'normal'?

✳ What is fulfilling and exciting for you?

Once you figure this out, think about what external factors are impacting it. Stress? Work? Relationships? Identifying these points is the first step towards addressing it.

How to talk about desire

So often, concerns around desire go unsaid. The person who desires sex less feels guilt for not giving their partner what they 'need', while the person who desires sex more feels guilty because they think they're expecting too much from their partner. It's really important that you don't make your partner feel like they are to blame, but it can also be super helpful to talk it out. It's often a personal and vulnerable conversation; treat each other with care.

Try these talking points:

✳ 'I've noticed we're not being sensual/sexual/playful with each other lately – have you noticed that too?'

✳ 'How do you currently feel in our relationship? Is there anything you'd like to prioritise more?'

✳ 'When do you desire sex most? I find I want sex when …'

✳ 'I feel sex is a really important part of our relationship and I want to make it better for us. Can we find a time to talk about it?'

✳ 'What are some sensual moments you'd like more of?'

Creating the ideal sexual context

Think about the ideal erotic equation for your sex life. What do you want and need more of in order to bring sex front of mind and make it feel like a priority again? Fill out the table below, using these prompts:

* How you feel emotionally, physically, sexually, etc.

* Location: home/holiday/locked door

* Types of touch/sex

* Specific qualities of sexual partners

* How you're feeling in relation to the person you're having sex with

* Anything else going on in your life.

Context for desire to thrive	Context for desire to fizzle

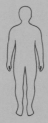

Engage your accelerators

As a two-week experiment, engage your accelerators every day for around ten minutes. That might mean a type of touch, something you do for yourself, something you do with someone else, erotica, masturbation, something you think about. This is all about creating more of a context for desire, and actively bringing pleasure front of mind. Notice how your body responds.

IMPORTANT STUFF

✳ Desire is one of the most common reasons people seek the support of a professional. It is normal to desire sex less or more than your partner, but if this is affecting your relationship, there's a lot you can do to work on this.

✳ It's useful for couples to understand the different ways they experience desire (spontaneous and responsive), as well as sharing what turns them on and off (and why) to create the context for desire.

✳ More often than not, it's the couples who prioritise playful and frequent sexual moments as a valuable part of their relationship (even when it's easier to watch a show in bed) who feel more connected, have more sex and are more fulfilled.

✳ If you're not prioritising sex, you need to make it pleasurable. That may mean taking penetration off the cards and coming back to what feels good: making out more, sensual massage, washing each other's bodies in the shower, telling your partner they look hot.

THE TECHNICAL STUFF

Techniques and positions for really, really good sex.

In this chapter you'll learn about dozens of different touch-based practices. These won't be pleasurable for everyone – just find what works for you. Use these as inspiration and build on them. The intention is to give you ideas, and hopefully a bit of confidence.

People often ask for my top hand and mouth tips and tricks. Of course I can offer you the fundamentals, though the best, most mind-blowing, failproof tip I can offer is this: *ask them what they like.* You could learn 41 different hand techniques and exercise your tongue muscles and train your gag reflex, but if you're in the role of 'giving pleasure' and you're not actually giving them what they enjoy, then every one of those 41 techniques will be useless. Ask them: 'How do you like to be touched? Licked? Sucked?' And if they don't know, you can explore together and learn. Ask them: 'What would make this even better? Would you like more or less pressure, speed, rhythm, vibration, movement, tongue, saliva, lube, etc.?' Be very descriptive with one another so you can figure out exactly what you like. There are heaps of ideas in here – you've got this!

Here are a few things to keep in mind while exploring techniques.

Slow the fuck down

I've said it a few times now: we're all having sex really quickly. That can be really fun, but starting slow is so useful. It gives you time to check in, build arousal, attune to your body and/or the other person's, and it also gives you more room to build intensity. Paring it back to start with can also be useful for when you feel overstimulated, when you're getting too aroused or it's not feeling so great. The same goes for intensity. Hard isn't always the best; it's often something to work up to.

Build arousal

Everything feels more intense when you're aroused. It's worth taking the time to touch, kiss and stimulate more than just the genitals (yes, this can even mean stimulating your brain to get you in the mood). Try full-body massage, breast or chest massage, moving to music, breathwork practices, external genital play, using toys around your body, erogenous zones, a meditation that brings awareness to your genitals, and literally anything else you like. Try teasing, brushing or hovering

over sensitive areas. This can do so much to build anticipation, leaving you yearning for the touch to return. Take your time to build arousal. And remember, we've got a whole chapter on foreplay.

Full-body touch

Your sexual partner is more than just their genitals. Awaken sensation in their whole body, kissing and touching them all over. Continue blended stimulation while you stimulate their genitals, as this is often the thing that can send them over the edge.

Five useful somatic tools

We can integrate these tools in any position or technique to add to our sexual experience: breath, movement, sound, touch and awareness.

Lube is always a good idea

Lube is a sex essential; it is the unsung hero of good sex. Its only purpose is to make sex feel really good for everyone. Sadly, there is shame and stigma around 'needing' to use it. But even if you were the wettest person in the world, sensitive external organs may never get the lubrication needed. Lube makes sex feel more comfortable, and can also make sex safer.

Create a sex toolkit

This can include anything from sex pillows, wedges, blindfolds, sensory items, toys, lube – anything to get your body in a comfortable position and allow you to access more pleasure.

Sex changes every time we do it

It's so exciting to learn tools, but it's also worth anticipating that a particular kind of touch may feel great one time and then kinda average the next. This is normal.

Check in with sexual partners

Refer to Chapters 7 and 8, on consent and communication. Asking your partner questions will help you nail touch far more effectively than a few illustrations in this book ever could.

The more present we feel, the better

It's clear from the thousands of conversations I've had about sex that the best and most memorable sex happens when we're feeling present and connected. Feeling present is a skill – see Chapter 2 for more on this.

Context is key

Context can make or break a good time; it's also pretty individual. It's important to consider what the other person might need to be able to release themselves into the experience. A locked door? The thrill of being caught? Making sure no one else is home? A new location? A clean room? Do what you can to ensure the context allows everyone to enjoy themselves.

Hygiene, taste and smell

Genitals will always smell and taste like genitals; they're not flowers. If you're feeling self-conscious about the way you taste or smell, the solution can be as simple as having a shower using a pH-balanced genital-safe wash to wash the penis and the vulva externally. Don't wash inside the vagina, however, as this can disrupt the pH balance. If you've had a long sweaty day or night, many people appreciate a sexual partner freshening up. This is also important because bacteria in the genitals or anus can enter the urethra during sex. Cleaning genitals before sex can reduce the risk of a UTI, as can peeing before and after sex. A shower can also help you relax and feel more comfortable giving and receiving.

If you do notice a serious change in the way your genitals smell or taste, or if there's an unusual odour, it's always best to see a doctor.

Hair

When it comes to body hair, my response is always the same: your body, your choice. You can never expect someone to trim, shape or remove pubic hair for your satisfaction, especially given that a choice around body hair is often personal, political or cultural. For some, hair may change the general experience of oral in that you may not have as easy access to sensitive areas. But making a judgement about someone's body is gross; don't do it.

If this is something you want to discuss with a partner, opt for curiosity over judgement, and be very comfortable with them telling you no. Celebrate their choice for their body. Shame or pressure should never be involved. Your partner may be willing to accommodate your wishes in some way, especially if it results in enhanced sensation, but remember, it's their body, and it's your responsibility to respect that.

Affirming identity and expression

If you're having sex with a trans, non-binary or gender-diverse person, celebrating and affirming their identity is crucial for a safe and positive experience. Use their pronouns and ask them how they like to refer to their genitals. For example, some trans men like their genitals to be referred to as a shaft or cock, and some trans women like their genitals to be referred to as their vulva, clit or pussy, but this isn't the case for everyone. If you don't know what someone calls their genitals, the best and most respectful thing to do is to ask.

It's useful for all people to share what they call their chest, genitals and body. This takes the onus off trans and gender diverse folk having to do all the leg work, and also acknowledges that we all have specific language we prefer, that feels more aligned to our bodies. This can also act as a turn-on. Acknowledge and celebrate your sexual partner, and continuously educate yourself about trans and non-binary experiences to deepen your understanding and empathy, because while it's useful for your partner to share their preferences, it can feel exhausting being the only source of education.

167

It's also worth noting that not all trans or non-binary individuals experience dysphoria (discomfort with one's body or gender-identity) during sex. While dysphoria is a valid and real experience for some, it is not universal. Sex and pleasure can also be transformative and healing. It can feel like a true experience of embodiment, especially when we recognise that pleasure is not limited to specific body parts or activities. Remember, if you've met one trans person, you've met one trans person. Everyone is different.

Sex and disability

People with disabilities have diverse sexual desires, needs and abilities, just like anyone else. Disability does not necessarily diminish someone's interest or desire for intimacy and pleasure. I don't specialise in sex and disability, but there are many practitioners, services, sex workers and providers who do.

I recommend checking out Bump'n and Luddi for tools, guides and resources. Before having sex, discuss any considerations that may make it a more pleasurable experience, set boundaries and get clear on any physical sensations or areas of sensitivity that you need to be aware of (this can include specific areas you or your partner do or don't want touched). Be patient and flexible, make use of tools and resources, check in, pause when you need to, and do whatever it is that you, as consenting, informed adults are willing and wanting to explore.

Focus on the experience

Yes, we love orgasms, but they're just a few seconds. Focusing on the whole experience of sex can feel so much greater than the peak moment of pleasure. Taking this approach helps everyone enjoy it more – giver and receiver.

Get comfortable; don't endure

To be a good giver, you need to be comfy! We don't want any sex injuries. If your back is sore, or you need to stretch out a cramp, do it. This is normal! Advocate for your comfort; doing so will help you focus and enjoy the experience.

Check in after

Aftercare is so important. Ask your partner how they'd like to integrate any sexual experience you've shared. Ask them what they liked, talk about what felt good, or what could be better.

Challenging sexual scripts

A sexual script is a blueprint of what we think we should do during sex. They are often a mainstream and rigid guideline for our expression, behaviour, desire and orientation, but we are not born with these scripts, they are learnt and are informed by socialisation. Through this sexual socialisation we learn how, who, when, where and why we are sexual, which can limit and restrict sexual expression and get in the way of us experiencing what we truly want. Though it may seem simple, journalling is a powerful tool to explore, process, understand yourself and integrate new learnings. For these reasons, practitioners commonly suggest journalling practices to support clients. Research has proven that journalling can lead to greater clarity and a better understanding of thoughts, fears and blockages as well as desires, and also promote autonomy and choice. See Chapter 1 for more prompts, reflective questions and activities.

Sex Positions

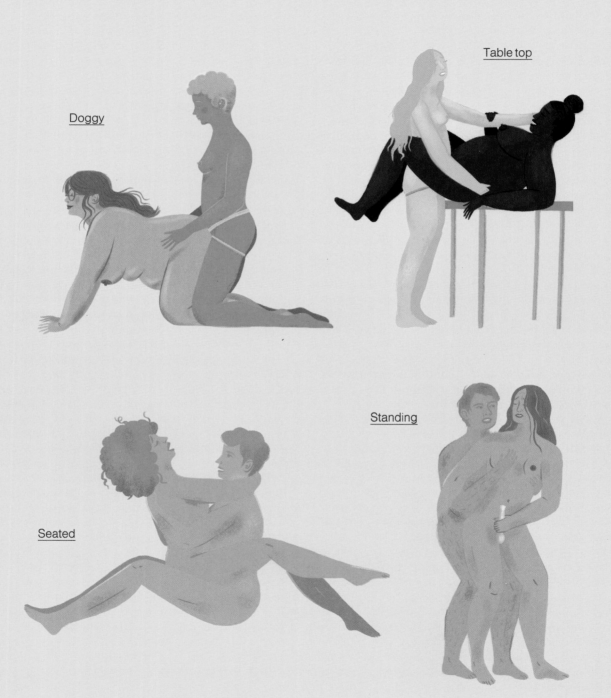

Table top

Doggy

Standing

Seated

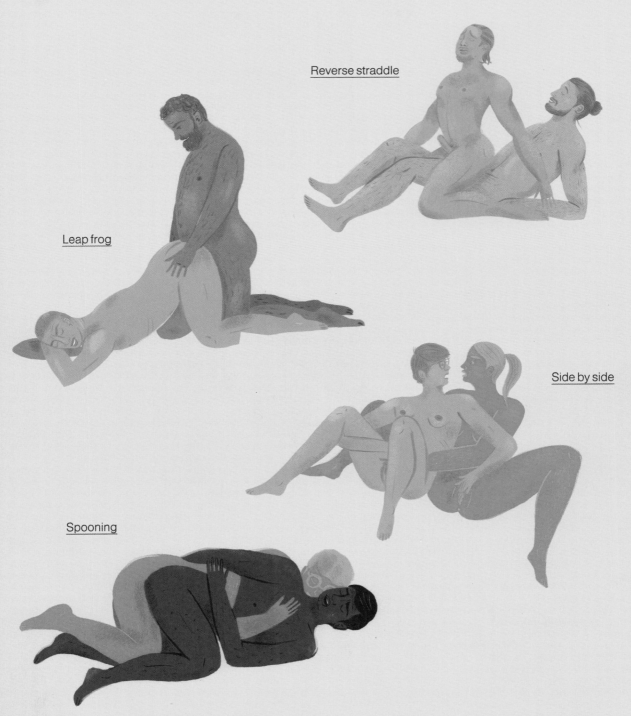

Reverse straddle

Leap frog

Side by side

Spooning

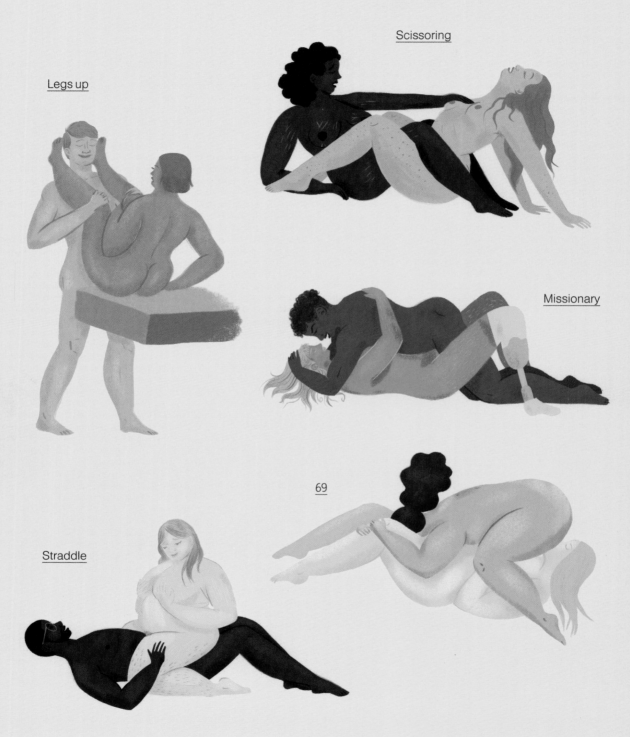

Scissoring

Legs up

Missionary

69

Straddle

SEX WITH A VULVA

Whether you have a vulva and/or you're having sex with someone with a vulva, or both, this section covers techniques for oral, fingering and penetrative sex. It's worth revisiting Chapter 4 to brush up on all the basics of anatomy, and, if you have a vulva, getting to know your own body first. The intention of this section is to really debunk the idea that vaginal penetration is the only way to have sex.

A quick note on clit sensitivity: some people love direct stimulation of the clit, while others find it too intense. It's all normal, but you'll need to ask, to ensure you give your partner a pleasurable experience, free from discomfort.

Oral

People always want to know how to improve their oral skills or to learn to receive so they can feel confident and enjoy it – and, honestly, go you. People with vulvas are statistically more likely to orgasm from acts like oral sex than penetrative sex, as they're receiving direct stimulation of the clit. When performing vulva-based oral sex, it's important to remember that there's a lot more to this part of the body than just the clitoris.

For a really great time, explore, experiment with and stimulate the whole vulva and rest of the body.

Set the mood

As mentioned towards the beginning of this chapter, it's important to take your time to build arousal. Relax into the moment and support your partner in receiving, awakening sensation in the whole body first.

Different ways to use your tongue

As a general rule, start slow and steady; you can always build the pace. Experiment with different styles of pressure and tongue motion, including:

✳ Using the flat, wide part of your tongue and running it all the way up the labia until you reach the glans of the clitoris (and beyond). You may choose to wiggle your tongue on the way up to stimulate the inner labia and clitoris. Pause to build anticipation, and then repeat.

✳ Moving your tongue up and down, left, right or in circles using a variety of speeds, rhythm and pace.

✳ Kissing the vulva, labia and clitoris with variation in pressure as you would lips. Don't be afraid to add a lil French kiss in there too.

✳ Sucking with your tongue and/or your lips at the same time, starting slowly to make sure they're into it.

✳ Using the tip of your tongue (the thinnest and strongest part) to apply direct pressure to the most arousing areas, then use your favourite directional stroke.

✳ Making your lips wet with saliva, then with your tongue inline with your lips move your mouth in a figure 8 direction from vaginal opening, across urethral opening, across then up and around the glans on the clit then back down to the vaginal opening. You can also get your nose to gently graze the clit and other sensitive areas.

Externally

Kiss, lick, tickle, tease and even use your breath on sensitive areas around their lower stomach and inner thighs. You can use your hands and mouth at the same time.

Outer labia

Kiss, lick and/or gently suck around the vulva without touching the external glands on the clit. Just kiss around the vulva to tease.

Inner labia

This is a really sensitive area. Start by gently using the tip of your tongue in an upwards direction, not yet touching the clit. You may also kiss the inner labia. With long, sweeping strokes, move your tongue from the vagina up to the clit. Start slowly and gently, then build intensity from there.

Clit

The clit is incredibly sensitive. Move the flat part of your tongue across the clit, either up and down or just up, moving your tongue in circles, either clockwise or anticlockwise. Try one of these techniques for a few rounds, rather than going through all of them at once. If your partner says they like it or they're giving you nonverbal cues that they're into it, stick with that technique for a while.

Vaginal opening

Concentrate on the vaginal opening, either circling your tongue around it, moving your tongue up and down, or pressing your tongue into the vagina to collect more lubrication and bring it up towards the clit. Press the flat part of your tongue on the opening, then slide the tongue upwards towards the clit. This sweeping motion accesses a lot of sensitive areas, from the vaginal opening, up towards the urethral opening, the bottom part of the clit and beyond.

Perineum

Occasionally licking or kissing this area in between stimulating the clit can add blended stimulation.

Maintain your rhythm

If they're about to climax, stay with the technique that is about to get them there. It's worth asking if they'd like more intensity or less. Some people want a face deep in their vulva going hard when they're cumming, while for others that would be way too sensitive. You'll need to ask them what they like.

Get your face into it

You can use more than just your tongue to create new sensations. Try using your lips (keep them wet so they slide over sensitive areas), your nose (let it gently move over the clit, urethral opening or vaginal opening), your breath (breathe cool or warm air onto their vulva). Think about it like you're making out with their vulva, try to tune into the rhythm, take it slow and see how their body responds.

What to do with your hands?

Sometimes you may need your hands and arms to prop yourself up, but at other times you can use them to stimulate the whole body, tickling nipples, gently scratching up and down the sides of their body, holding their bum, hips or legs, if they're into it. Try stimulating other erogenous zones with touch.

Fingering or penetrating the vagina

Stimulating the vagina at the entrance can be enough to make some people climax. Others may want to be penetrated with a come here motion, in and out penetration or thrusting. Refer to the fingering tips on pages 177–178.

Positions for going down

* Receiver has their legs open wide, giver is lying in between their legs.

* Receiver has their legs bent up, giver is lying in between their legs.

* 69: Both bodies are giving and receiving, facing each other simultaneously going down.

* Receiver is seated with legs open, giver is kneeling between their legs.

* Face sitting: Receiver is hovering, squatting or sitting on giver's face.

* Kivin method: Receiver is lying on their back, giver is lying perpendicular and stimulating the vulva from the side – so it kinda looks like a T shape.

PRO TIPS FOR GREAT ORAL SEX

You don't need to fit this all into one sesh; sometimes less is more. Start with a few of these techniques and positions and see what they like.

⁕ To ensure there's enough lubrication, make sure your lips are wet and that there's a layer of saliva on your tongue. Some may not want too much saliva as they may not like the feeling of it dripping down to their anus. It's often a goldilocks moment to figure out the perfect amount.

⁕ Affirm them while you're going down on them. Tell them that you like the way they taste, moan as you lick, remind them you'll tell them if you need to pause.

⁕ Using sound, such as moaning, can add more vibration.

⁕ Use a toy internally or externally while you lick, kiss or suck.

⁕ Tease. When intensity builds, move away or pause with your tongue on the clitoris, then return to their favourite stroke. Taking breaks throughout to kiss their outer labia or legs can build anticipation and arousal, making them yearn for more touch.

⁕ For more anticipation and sensation play, keep their underwear on and work your way around it, starting outside on the inner thighs and outer labia, then working your way in.

⁕ Experiment with speed. You'd be surprised by how good it can feel when you're going really slowly, building to a crescendo or sticking to a deliberate rhythm.

Fingering

Prep your hands; make sure you have clean, smooth and short nails. The vagina has a microbiome of its own, and we want to protect it from any unwanted guests – a quick hand wash never goes astray. Lube is also a great idea – the majority of people experience greater pleasure and comfort with a little (body-safe) lubricant. It's worth noting that a lot of these techniques can be used for solo or partnered sex.

The clitoris is sensitive to variations in stroking, pressure and rhythm. With plenty of lubrication, try the following:

External stimulation

✳ **Warm up:** Start with the palm cupping the vulva and stroke upwards towards the stomach, softly playing with the clit on the way. After a while, move your fingers between the labia, even placing the pad of the finger on the vaginal opening.

✳ **Tapping:** Try a gentle and slow tapping motion of the clit and clitoral hood, experimenting with speed, rhythm and pressure. You could remove touch entirely, or keep touch connected and add more pressure.

✳ **Circles:** A crowd fave! In a circular motion, move your fingers across the most sensitive and pleasurable parts of the clit. This may mean stroking around the clit or directly stimulating it.

✳ **Motion:** Using your fingers, rub up and down, or side to side across the clitoris. Check in regularly: *What pressure, rhythm or sensations are feeling really good?*

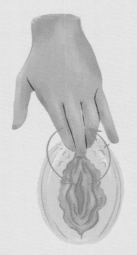
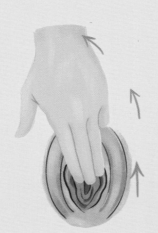
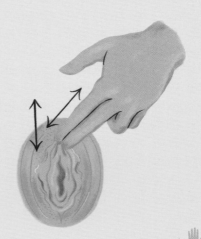

Internal stimulation

As you're trying these techniques, keep asking your partner questions: *How many fingers? What kind of motion? Is that the G-spot!?*

✳ **Come hither:** Press one or two fingers into the G-spot inside the vagina (see Chapter 4 if you're not sure where it is) and motion forward, towards your palm, as if you're beckoning someone to come closer. With the right amount of pressure, come hither can lead to squirting (more on this later in the chapter!).

✳ **Windscreen wiper:** Curl your fingers and move them from side to side across the G-spot in a swiping motion while inside the vagina.

✳ **Penetrating:** Starting with your fingers at the entrance, thrust them in and out to the depth that's most pleasurable. Rub your fingers across the front wall of the vagina, then bring them out towards the entrance and repeat.

✳ **Thudding:** This is basically penetrating, but the base of the fingers/knuckles makes more of an impact on the vaginal opening.

✳ **Double time:** With your palm facing the vulva, use the base of your hand to stimulate the clitoris up and down, while your middle fingers stay inside the vagina, moving with the 'come hither' motion.

✳ **Triple time:** Adding to double time, with two fingers inside massaging the G-spot, palm on the clit, use your other hand to cup or massage the perineum, anus or bum for further stimulation. Alternatively, use your other hand to play with their nipples.

✳ **Fisting:** This is the act of penetrating someone with your whole hand. The name of this technique is kind of misleading in that you're not (necessarily) penetrating them with a closed fist – instead, the fingers are kept straight and closely grouped together to kinda look like you're making a duck beak with your hand. This can feel really good for anyone who likes feeling full.

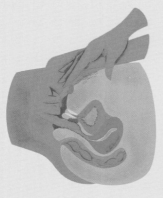
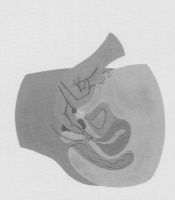
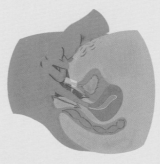

Important note: when you or they want to stop internally stimulating, pull your fingers or hand out slowly (unless they tell you otherwise). Some people also like to have their vulva cupped by the hand that was just penetrating them; this can add a sense of safety and comfort.

Stimulating someone else's G-spot

The G-spot is kind of similar to a penis in that this erectile tissue engorges and becomes erect with arousal. Start by building arousal (refer to the information at the start of this chapter), then when they're feeling aroused and want internal stimulation, insert your finger with your fingertips facing the front wall of their body.

To find the sensitive area, you'll probably only need to insert your fingers to about the second knuckle (though this is different for everyone), then hook them around with a 'come hither' motion. If they're not aroused, the G-spot will feel slightly rough and ridgey – kind of like the roof of your mouth. It could even be uncomfortable to touch. If that's the case, slow it right down. If they are aroused, it should feel more supple and soft, almost like the inside of your cheek (try running your tongue across the inside of your cheek to feel). If you're looking to really

increase pleasure here, I'd introduce a toy of some kind for external stimulation of the clitoris and/or vulva.

Positions

Vaginal sex isn't the only way to have sex, but we're flooded with imagery about it in our culture, sex ed and porn. It's often the default mode for having sex, but let's not forget, it's just one way to do it. A quick Google search will offer you infinite positions to try. While it's always great to be open to trying new things, sometimes all you need are a few staple positions that feel good for all bodies involved, then you can add extra stimulation from there. A lot of these positions are dependent on the body and anatomical make-up, and what feels accessible to you, so you'll need to do some exploration. You can try any of these while including fingers, vibrators and, of course, lube. Lots and lots of lube.

✳ **Missionary:** Face to face and on top of each other.

✳ **Seated/reverse seat:** One person on a seat, person with vulva sitting on top, either facing their partner or facing away.

* **Straddle:** I'm rebranding this from cowgirl/cowboy for a more gender neutral option. One person sits on top and straddles the other, and can either face their partner or face away from them.

* **Doggy:** Either on all fours or bum in the air, higher than shoulders, being penetrated from behind.

* **On top/on bottom:** Switch between being on top or on the bottom, legs and bodies in a variety of configurations.

* **Legs up:** One or two legs in the air, while someone holds them up, or rests the legs on their shoulders.

* **Face down:** Either lying down with legs straight or one slightly cocked out.

* **Pretzel:** The penetrating partner straddles the receiving partner's leg, with the other one over their shoulder; it can also be lying down or bent.

COMMON QUESTIONS ABOUT SQUIRTING

What is it? The truth is, there's still a lot we don't know about squirting, as there's not a lot of conclusive evidence. Ejaculating, squirting and gushing are pleasurable experiences that are not related to vaginal lubrication, as these fluids are expressed out the urethral opening when you're aroused. Despite what porn will have you believe, squirting doesn't necessarily happen at the peak of orgasm; it can happen before, during or after orgasm. But it can feel like an intense release. The terms ejaculating, squirting and gushing are used interchangeably, but some research suggests they are different. Ejaculate has a milky, cum-like consistency and can look similar to what a penis ejaculates. Squirt can look more watery and can sometimes have ejaculate in it, while gushing is different in the amount that is expressed – sometimes it can be enough to soak the bed.

Can everyone do it? Everyone with a vulva has the mechanics to do it, but this doesn't necessarily mean they will or that they want to. There are only small studies on these areas, so we don't have a realistic figure, though one study found that 69.23 per cent of participants experienced ejaculation during orgasm.

Isn't it just wee? I'm less concerned with proving it's not wee and more concerned with supporting people to feel comfortable with their body expressing fluids during sex. Sex involves fluids, cum, sweat, sometimes tears, sometimes menstrual blood and sometimes squirt. There is still no conclusive agreement among scientists as to what the fluid actually is. A penis can cum and wee out of the same tube, so why is it so hard to believe that people with vulvas can do this too? Some studies have found that ejaculate fluid contains traces of urine and may also contain a combination of other fluids. Other research suggests that the fluid is expressed out of the Skene's glands, which are secretory glands located near the urethra. Interestingly, they've found ejaculate to be mostly prostate enzymes with a small percentage of urea, whereas squirting is diluted urine with a small percentage of ejaculate in it. Sex is messy, let's embrace it.

Note: During sexual arousal, the Skene's glands, two small ducts on either side of the urethra, swell as blood flows to the genital region, and secrete a milky fluid throughout sex and potentially at peak moments of pleasure. This fluid contains similar proteins to those found in penile ejaculation.

Some researchers believe the Skene's glands are the source of ejaculation in people with vulvas.

How can I learn to do it? Good news: the best way to learn how to squirt is to masturbate, and masturbate often. Sometimes it's easier using toys or having someone else stimulate you, as it can be tricky to add direct stimulation.

✳ **The more relaxed and aroused you are, the better:** When you're practising squirting, you're learning to let go of hard-wired patterns of clenching your pelvic floor. It may take time to relax and release into the moment. Do what you can to relax and release your pelvic floor.

Note: you may want to wee before you try this, and empty your bladder entirely to create a sense of ease and a reminder that you're not actually wetting the bed.

✳ **Clitoral stimulation:** This is really important – as we've addressed, the G-spot is part of the clitoral network, so it's really useful to stimulate your clit.

🖐 181

* **Stimulate your G-spot:** While you masturbate externally, insert your fingers, facing up, to massage the G-spot. The more aroused you are, the more engorged the G-spot will be, so wait until you're turned on to find it. You can use your fingers or a curved G-spot toy to locate your G-spot and massage it. Some people find G-spot stimulation deeply pleasurable, others don't – there's nothing wrong with you if it's not your thing! Try thudding rather than rubbing, Thudding is a deeper, more repetitive pressure on the front side of the vaginal wall. Repetition in this way can stimulate a feeling of 'build up', which can then lead to the sense that you're going to wee.

* **Listen to your body:** If you feel you're about to wee, don't worry – you've already emptied your bladder. This is a sign you may be close to squirting! Relax and release your pelvic floor, lengthen your exhale, start thrusting your hips and follow the pleasure.

* **Practise!** It may take a bit of practice – the good news is, it'll be pleasurable homework. Remember: take the goal out of sex and prioritise pleasure instead.

Deeper penetration

Many people love receiving deep vaginal penetration as this may hit the A-spot (anterior fornix), an erogenous zone of sensitive tissue up near the cervix, as well as the cervix itself. Every vagina is a different length, so some people may be able to reach the A-spot with their fingers while others can't. This is where a toy, dildo or vibrator can come in handy. Stimulating this part of the body can be incredibly pleasurable and feel really great. Remember that you don't need to jump in straight away, and that most sexual experiences can be enhanced simply by taking the time to turn yourself (or your partner) on.

Vulva-on-vulva sex

Porn, limited sex education, and the heteronormative expectations that exist today have affected the way we understand vulva-on-vulva sex. And that goes for people who do it, people who want to do it and people who just want to know more about it. It's important to remember that sex means different things for different people; no two sexual experiences will be the same. I should also point out that a lot of this book will set you up for great vulva-on-vulva sex – after all, it's sex with someone else, and by now you're fully prepped for great sex with someone else. Also, you have a similar anatomy, and while you might not like the same things, you have prior knowledge from exploring your own body.

Scissoring

Many people are familiar with 'scissoring', and will often assume it's the position of choice for vulva-on-vulva sex. While scissoring can feel really good, it is just one way to have sex. The word 'scissoring' is used interchangeably with 'tribbing', which essentially means two people rub, hump or thrust their vulvas or bodies together.

This is a position that is largely misunderstood, so it's important to know a few things:

* Not everyone likes to scissor.

* Not all people get off from scissoring.

* It can be incredibly pleasurable, orgasmic, intimate and hot.

* Not just lesbians scissor. Anyone can try it, and you don't need two vulvas.

* You can scissor with more than just genitals – try humping legs, arms, bums, stomachs, pillows.

* Scissoring may include penetration, but it also may not.

* Safer-sex practices are still needed, as genitals may be involved.

* Toys will add new sensations; for example, a palm vibe between bodies.

Using strap-ons and sex toys

Wearing a strap-on can be fun, deeply sensual and hot. Not all vulva-on-vulva sex includes strap-ons. If you're curious about trying them but unsure where to start, let's take it right back to basics.

183

* **Do your own research:** It's important to do your research and get a sense of what strap-ons suit you and your needs. Look for style, material, comfort, O-ring size (the hole you put the dildo through), size of harness and whether you want adjustable straps. You may want a harness or you may opt for underwear that has an O hole in it, which comes in a range of styles, including options that are more masc or femme so you can play with embodying the strap-on that feels best suited to you.

* **Try it on:** Try it outside of a sexual experience and get used to how it feels on your body. Many of my clients without penises love the feeling, the look, and how they can embody a new side of them. Try walking around with it, dancing, thrusting, or even masturbating with the strap-on. This can also help you get used to it, as the dildo isn't a part of your body. Sometimes it can feel like it moves around; this is normal, and with a bit of practice you'll get used to it.

* **Think about how/when you want to use it:** Is it for you to wear, or for someone else? Is it for vaginal, anal or oral? What does an exciting sexual experience look like? Be clear on your interests, curiosities and concerns.

* **Discuss with your partner:** This should happen before, during and after all sexual experiences, particularly when you're trying something new. Ask them if you're going too deep or not deep enough, how the material feels on their skin, and tell them how it feels for you. It may take time to get used to wearing it, but communication will help you learn together. This goes for every new person you try it with.

* **Practise:** Like any new skill, it may take you time to get into the groove. That's okay! Practise by yourself or create a practice and play session with others.

* **Sex positions:** Try any of the sex positions detailed earlier in this chapter. Often it can feel easier if the person being penetrated starts on top so that they can set the speed, pace and rhythm. The person who's wearing the strap-on can also hold the dildo in place if they need. This is an individual preference. A position like missionary, where your hands are free, can be a great place to start. But if you're pegging anally or if you want to thrust on your knees, the receiver may choose to start on all fours so the giver can get a good grip.

* **Take care of it:** Follow the care and cleaning instructions, and practise safer sex with your strap-on. These tools are an investment, and if you take care of them, they'll last longer.

Common misconceptions

Just because two people with vulvas are having sex doesn't mean they're both lesbians. They could be pansexual, queer, bisexual, heterosexual ... They may also not be cis women – they may be trans women, non-binary, genderfluid. The only way to 'tell' someone's sexuality is if they freely tell you without feeling pressured.

Myth: *One is always the man*

Truth: Asking a lesbian couple or two people who have vulvas *who's the man, who wears the pants, who pays for dinner, who holds the door open* is an insight into heterosexual expectations penetrating queer dynamics. This may be true for some relationships, but it certainly isn't the only structure to a relationship. When someone asks this, it actually reveals more about the way they have sex – they can only imagine sex as a penis penetrating a vagina.

Myth: *Straight men are allowed to watch*

Truth: I can't tell you how many times cis men have asked me this and it's fucking creepy. If you have the thought, that's totally fine – our minds often wander to sexy and/or disturbing places. But please, dear god, don't say them out loud to a stranger or someone you're not in a flirty/sexual dynamic with.

SEX WITH AN ANUS

We've all got an anus and there's a hole lot to be experienced here (sorry, I had to). Anal sex can feel pleasurable, orgasmic and incredibly relaxing. People of all sexualities and genders are into anal, because it feels so damn good! There's lots of pleasurable nerve endings and erectile tissue in the anus – in fact, the anus has the second highest concentration of nerve endings in your body (the clit is no. 1). Someone once told me their first anal orgasm was the most intense, full-body and emotionally intimate experience they've ever had.

Why does it feel so good?

Anal orgasms can feel different for everyone, and each time you have them. Some describe an anal orgasm as:

✳ intense waves of pleasure that begin deep inside your body

✳ a pulse of contractions

✳ a full-body release

✳ a deeply relaxing experience

✳ an intimate, connecting, sensual, vulnerable practice.

People with penises say it feels like an ejaculatory orgasm, just way more intense. Some people like anal sex or stimulation on its own, while others like it as part of wider sexual experiences. The bottom line? It may not be for everyone, but it can feel like some of the most intense and pleasurable sex you'll ever have. All people can climax from anal sex.

Relaxation, clean and prep

As with all sex, the more relaxed you are, the better it feels. There's so much you can try when building arousal for anal sex.

✳ **Anal breathing practices:** Don't worry, I'm not suggesting your anus has a different set of lungs. Anal breathing is just about engaging your anus on an inhale and releasing it on an exhale. This sounds so simple, but it can have an immediate physiological effect on your body. When you hold your breath (as many people do during sex) the whole body stiffens and the anus tightens up. Tensing the entire body, including squeezing the anus, is directly linked to stress. Mindful or 'anal' breathing will not only calm your nervous system, it will also invite sensation into your body, relax your anus and allow for deeper pleasure.

✳ **Releasing tension:** Everyone walks around with their bum clenched; you might even notice you're clenching while reading this. Actively try to release tension in your glutes on a regular basis, but particularly during sex.

✳ **Daily anal massage in the shower:** Keep a nice oil or silicon-based lube in the shower for a daily massage to get comfortable with exploring pleasure on a daily basis.

✳ **Anal massage:** There are a few techniques on how to do this for someone else later in this chapter; you can also start by practising this touch on your own first.

How to prep for anal

If anal sex is something you want to try, or is something you're having regularly, there are some really basic things you can do to feel safe, clean, prepped and relaxed. It really doesn't need to be a big ordeal though. We all have different things we do to feel good going into sex, the same goes for anal. Some choose to do a lot of prep and some do very little.

✳ **The lifestyle approach:** You may hear jokes about Metamucil being your bestie, but really this is just about eating a high-fibre diet so you can empty your bowels before you do anal. Or it might be that you opt out of anal sex if you've had a big, spicy meal or you've eaten ice cream and you're lactose intolerant. But you really don't need to change your diet or lifestyle.

✳ **The low-maintenance approach:** Simply using baby wipes or damp toilet paper to feel extra fresh. You could have a quick shower and manually clean your anus externally and/or internally with a finger.

✳ **The deep-clean approach:** This involves investing in an enema or douche, but it's best to clean up 1 to 2 hours prior if you're going for this deeper clean, just in case you stimulate the digestive system. Make sure you follow the instructions on how to use the enema or douche safely.

✳ **The squeaky-clean approach:** If you're really concerned about hygiene, wearing gloves can be a cleaner (and, hey, kinkier) option.

Safer sex is sexy, so I'd also recommend wearing condoms and, importantly, never move directly from anal to other genitals or the mouth. Ever. Instead, make sure you thoroughly clean whatever you're using – be it a toy, hand or genitals – with water and a genital-safe body wash or a toy cleaner. Transferring the bacteria from anus to vagina can cause serious problems. When you want to switch it up, remove and change the condom, and make sure you've washed whatever's been in the rectum with genital-safe soap and water before switching to vaginal sex. If you don't want to have to pause in between, you can always save anal till the end.

TALK ABOUT IT

Just like trying anything new, it's important to have the conversation before you're in the heat of the moment. It can feel particularly awkward or clunky asking for something that has a cultural and societal judgement around it. If you want to try exploring anal sex or stimulation but you're struggling to bring it up, it may be worth reading this chapter with your partner. Or saying something like, 'Hey, I'm curious about anal pleasure; how would you feel about trying it together?' They may want more information, like whether they'll be giving or receiving, penetrating or being penetrated, and the type or style of sex you're curious about. They may be into it, and they may not. If it's not their thing, it can still be yours during solo sex. This conversation doesn't just happen before sex – you need to keep the communication up during and after, too! Check out Chapter 8 for tips on how best to do this.

Many people say they feel intimidated by anal play as a result of their social conditioning, limited sex education or simply an ingrained belief that the bum has only one function (and I'm not referring to anal breathing). I'd always recommend starting with yourself so you can get to know your own body and your own limits. There are two types of anal play: external and internal. These don't all involve climax or penetration, but rather they are a bunch of different ways you can have or give really pleasurable experiences.

Fingering

External

✳ **The doorbell:** Press the pad of your thumb or finger on the anus. This is a great technique for beginners, because when you're using the flat part of your thumb or finger it can feel reassuring to know that it's not going to be inserted. Explore rhythm, pace, tapping and pressure as you stimulate the anus.

✳ **Mapping:** Mapping is a great practice that is all about locating or mapping out different sensations in your anus (although, really, you can do this over your whole body). As you explore pressure, speed and rhythm, you may find areas that are pleasurable, and you may find areas that feel numb. Depending on your enquiry, be it for pleasure or exploration, you may use different types of touch to bring pleasure or awareness to your anus.

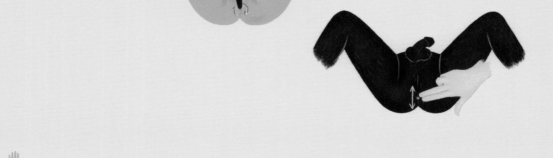

* **Stroking:** Using any finger, stroke the anus in an up or down direction.

* **Circles:** With an index finger, massage the rim of the anus with a circular motion. Play with different pressure, circle size and speed.

* **Twinkle, twinkle:** Using two hands, cup the bum cheeks and walk your fingers up and down the anus as if you were playing scales on a piano. Like all good musicians, explore and experiment with different variations in touch.

* **Swipe:** Using the pinky side of your hand, swipe it between the bum cheeks, up and down with plenty of lube. This kinda looks like swiping a credit card through a machine (before we were all tapping). You may even bring some vibration or movement to your hand as you swipe it through.

Internal

It's really important that you take time to build arousal through external anal play, as this makes internal stimulation feel so much better. If your partner's anus is really tight, it's always best to focus on external stimulation. Don't push through pain or discomfort. Often the anus winks, or opens and closes, when it's really relaxed, making it more comfortable and pleasurable to penetrate.

* **Come hither:** Fingers face upwards in a 'come here' motion to stimulate sensitive areas.

* **Prostate massage:** This is for someone with a penis/prostate. With lube, gently insert your finger curving towards the front of the body. About two inches in, you'll find the prostate, which will feel smooth and round like a plum. Try a range of motions: 'come here', pressing, penetrating or rubbing with your fingers while also experimenting with pressure, speed or rhythm. As one of the most pleasurable areas, the prostate swells during arousal, making it easier to find.

* **Penetrating:** In and out movement, thrusting, play with pressure and rhythm.

* **Toys:** Plugs, prostate massager, anal beads (more on these options in Chapter 14).

* **Blended:** Stimulate other erogenous zones – clit, nipples, penis, etc.

Rimming/oral

Also called analingus, rimming is orally stimulating the anus with your tongue and mouth. Just like any other form of oral sex, rimming can feel really pleasurable, sexy and intimate. It's important to check in before you stick your tongue between the cheeks. Make sure your partner is into it or curious about it.

Start building arousal by kissing their bum and gently licking between the cheeks, then use your tongue to stimulate the anus. Try circles, up and down, side to side, pressure, blowing hot or cool air or even teasing with external vibration in between oral stimulation. If you're interested in this but don't want to put your tongue into the anus, a dental dam can come in handy. As always, safer-sex practices are important. Condoms and dental dams are the best way to minimise your risk of STIs, and they can also provide a sexy physical barrier for any tongue and bum play.

Positions

Take your time to tease, stimulate, and build arousal of your whole body. When you're both turned on and ready, you can move to some external anal stimulation (see the previous sections). Remember to start slow, then slow it down even more. When it feels good, play around with speed and rhythm.

* **Face down:** Lie face down with your arms by your sides or make a hand cushion for your forehead, with your legs slightly apart. The penetrating partner kneels behind you or lies on top of you, in between your legs.

* **Missionary:** Face to face and on top of each other.

* **Legs up:** Lie on your back, knees towards your chest, holding them with your hands. The penetrating partner can kneel in front of you to massage or penetrate.

* **On side:** Lie on your side. Bring your outer leg towards your chest, with your partner behind you to reach your anus.

* **Doggy:** On all fours with your partner behind you. Some people like to stretch their arms forward so their bum is higher than their shoulders.

* **Standing:** One person in front of the other. The person in front may want to hold on to something or bend over slightly.

Accessorise

Get your sexual toolkit and come prepared. It's really important to use a good-quality lube, condoms and even a few toys. You can use vibrators, butt plugs, anal beads and glass dildos. If you are inserting a toy, it MUST MUST MUST have a flared base – there have been all too many cases of objects getting lodged inside the body. A flared base will keep you safe. Good-quality, body-safe lubes and toys will help build arousal and awareness of your anus, two very important things to do before any penetration.

Numbing creams

Many people use numbing creams for anal penetration, but I do not recommend this. Pain is there to tell you when you're pushing your body too far, and sex should never involve unwanted pain. If you're consistently having painful sex and needing to numb yourself, I would recommend trying these instead:

✳ Slowing down and building arousal first, before jumping into penetration.

✳ Exploring different types of foreplay, like anal massage, rimming and external stimulation.

✳ Changing to a position where you feel like you have more control on the depth of penetration.

✳ ALWAYS telling your partner if you're experiencing pain. Try saying something like:

   ✳ 'Let's pause and try a different angle.'

   ✳ 'I'd like to control the pace and depth this time so I can make sure it feels comfortable.'

   ✳ 'I need to slow down, this doesn't feel great.'

   ✳ 'Can we try this now? I'm in pain.'

   ✳ 'Let's start slow this time, I want to build arousal first.'

   ✳ 'Last time it was uncomfortable/ painful, and I want to do things differently from now on.'

✳ Seeking professional support – it may be useful to speak with your doctor, a sex therapist or a sexologist if pain continues beyond all of this.

POPPERS/AMYL

Colloquially referred to as poppers, inhaled nitrite is a liquid drug that gives a high, spaced out, dizzy feeling when you inhale it. Poppers are also used in penetrative anal sex to relax the anal sphincters. Although they are widely used, that doesn't necessarily mean they're the best thing for your body. They can have dangerous side effects and can be fatal. Using poppers is risky, and the high is only very short, so it is best not to use them. There are many other ways to relax the anus for pain-free and pleasurable anal sex – check out the ideas on the previous pages.

More than just penetration

Anal sex is for anyone. With the right prep, lots of lube, checking in, tuning in to your body and other people's bodies, it can be the best sex of your life. When it comes to anal sex, remember that this isn't just about shoving it in and going for it. Anal sex can be so much more than penetration, and it should be enjoyable for everyone involved. If it's not feeling good, stop, pause or reassess. Experiment with toys, try out external and internal play, and unpack the myths about what anal sex means or what it should be. Really, it's whatever you make it; hot, intense, deeply intimate, connective, full body, orgasmic.

Common misconceptions

Myth: It's gay

Truth: There's a lot to unpack here – the belief that anal is 'gay sex', and that if you enjoy a body part or toy in your rectum, that proves something about your sexual identity. I've even heard of people feeling uncomfortable washing their bum in the shower, fearful of their own hand near their anus. So let's be clear here: liking anal sex doesn't say anything about your sexuality. Imagine assuming this about any other

erogenous zone. *You like your neck being kissed; you must be bisexual.* Your anus is an erogenous zone, and it can feel really good. The only thing that determines your sexual identity is you – not a body part that you like having touched. If you've ever thought anal is gay, it'll be useful to examine, challenge and unpack any internalised homophobia within yourself and reflect on why you're not touching a particular body part.

Myth: It's messy

Truth: Anal does not have to be a messy experience, and more often than not, it isn't. With a bit of awareness and some really simple preparation, you can completely minimise mess and feel sexy the whole time. Flick back to page 186 if you need a reminder.

Myth: It will hurt

Truth: Unless pain is something that you or your partner is actively engaging in (i.e. spanking), sex should never be painful. Anal sex is all about pleasure.

Myth: It's only hard and fast fucking

Truth: There's so much more to anal than hard and fast penetration. Sure, many people love having anal in this way, but this is just one way to have anal sex. As we've discussed throughout this chapter, anal sex can involve toys, fingers and penises. It can be sexy, sensual and intimate.

SEX WITH A PENIS

Whether you have a penis, you have sex with a penis, or both, this section will work to expand your knowledge of pleasure. We have a very limited idea of what sex with a penis can look like. These limits leave out a lot of nuance, and also place a lot of pressure on someone with a penis to perform in the way that porn stars do. We're often socialised to think that people with penises are simple and people with vulvas are complex. There's an assumption that people with penises don't want or need context, setting, safety, communication or time to build arousal, that they're predictable and ready to go at any time.

This is bullshit, and inaccurate. I have worked extensively with people with penises and men, and they are just as in need of all of these things. This doesn't make them any less of a man, it makes them human. We've already seen in Chapter 4 how similar the structure of the penis and clit are. Sure, the penis hangs

outside of the body while the majority of the clit is inside the body, but these body parts are more similar than they are different. Many people with penises don't just want to 'get it up and get it in'. Yes, of course, this can be hot for some, but not for everyone. If we want to change the way we have sex for all people, we need to acknowledge how sexual scripts affect us all.

Oral

There's a bit of a formula to giving great head. After speaking with many people who both give and receive blow jobs, I've put together the following list of things to keep in mind.

Go slow

Take your time to build arousal, without rushing or diving into a deep throat. Try awakening sensation all over the body with a solid dose of foreplay – kissing, consistent touch, dirty talk, a slow lick/ kiss down the chest, lower stomach and thighs. Here, we're looking for teasing and building arousal, but not directly touching the shaft.

Tongue technique

Typically, the most sensitive part of the penis is its glans/head, particularly the frenulum. These are the areas that will feel the most pleasure when sucked or licked. Start by running your tongue from base to tip, experimenting with pressure and speed, sucking, kissing or creating a gentle vacuum with your mouth around the penis.

Techniques to try

✳ **Frenulum (the banjo string):** Start with soft and slow strokes with a relaxed tongue. Try licking, kissing or wrapping your whole mouth around the head of the penis while putting more pressure on the frenulum.

✳ **Glans/head:** The head or glans of the penis is really sensitive, so even a light touch can feel good. Gently suck, kiss and graze with your lips.

✳ **Shaft:** Wrap your mouth around the shaft, using either hand to stroke, with added tongue pressure on the frenulum. The shaft of the penis is less sensitive than the head, so it can feel good to add a bit more pressure, but always start slow and work your way up.

✳ **Base:** This area tends to be responsive to massage, with slow, mid-pressure stimulation. For example, if you're giving someone head, you might use one hand to massage the base of their penis while you use your tongue to stimulate the head and shaft.

✳ **Balls:** Testicles are sensitive – even gently cupping, ticking, pulling or holding can elicit a wave of pleasure. But go gently – using too much pressure without building your way up to it can be painful or uncomfortable.

✳ **Perineum:** This on its own can feel incredibly pleasurable – try licking, sucking or kissing it – but you can also add blended stimulation while giving head by massaging, kneading, tapping or using vibration on the gooch.

✳ **Prostate:** While giving head, try internal anal stimulation using a 'come here' motion, pressure or thrusting.

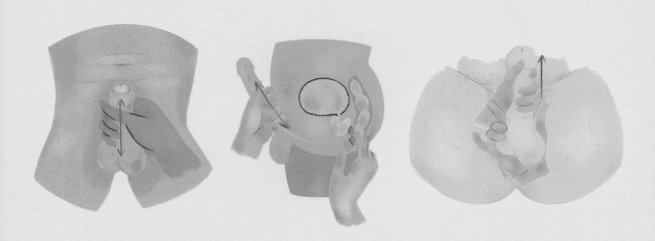

Deep throating

There's an assumption that in order to be good at head you have to deep throat. But blow jobs do not have to involve deep penetration in order to feel good. If you don't enjoy deep throating, if it's uncomfortable or you have a gag reflex, don't do it. If you want to incorporate more of the shaft, you can do this by using your hands or tongue up and down the shaft.

A gentle reminder that everyone receives pleasure in different ways. The best blow job you'll ever give is by learning about what your partner wants to receive. Keep an open line of dialogue around what your partner does/doesn't enjoy and what they want more/less of. This can be reviewed before, during or in those essential aftercare moments.

Wet 'n' wild

Generally, the wetter the better. Make sure you have enough saliva in your mouth to properly lubricate whatever part of the penis you're pleasuring. If in doubt, try a non-flavoured, body-safe lube to get the ball(s) rolling.

Edging

Edging is the practice of moving closer to orgasm, then stopping/pausing/slowing before reaching the point of no return. You can play with speed, rhythm and pressure to tease and bring your partner close to a climactic moment, then slow it down until they're ready to cum.

PRO-TIPS FOR GIVING GREAT HEAD

⁕ **Eye contact**: This can feel intense but intimate, sensual and sexy.

⁕ **Moaning**: This can really turn someone on. It also adds vibrations to the penis and stimulates it more intensely.

⁕ **Ball play**: Don't forget the testicles or perineum, which are both super-sensitive and erogenous zones. A lot of people love having their balls played with/nibbled/sucked.

⁕ **Handy**: Try using a combination of hands, lips and tongue to create a variety of pressure and sensation. Or suck on the balls while working the shaft with your hands. Try using a pepper grinder motion with your hands while rubbing your tongue on the underside of the head.

⁕ **Deep throat**: This means taking most of the penis in your mouth until it reaches the back of your throat. This isn't for everyone, and it certainly isn't essential. Take it slow, remember to breathe and take breaks whenever you need.

⁕ **Harmonica**: It doesn't all have to go in the mouth – try mouthing along the shaft like a harmonica, paying extra attention to the frenulum.

⁕ **Body language**: Read it – you may notice hip thrusts when it's feeling good, or tension or pulling back if it hurts.

⁕ **You might get messy**: A messy blow job and a lot of saliva can help your mouth glide over sensitive areas – don't be afraid to get sloppy!

⁕ **Try not to overthink it**: Treat head like a good make-out session.

⁕ **Have fun**: Consistently, people will share that head feels better when they know their partner is into it and wants to be doing it, so do things that feel good for your mouth too.

Hand jobs

Giving someone a hand job can be an art form. While some people are happy to stick with what feels good, others like a variety of grip strengths and stroke speeds. Sticking to the same strokes means you might be leaving out a range of erogenous zones. Here's what you should keep in mind:

* **Watch and learn:** A good way to learn is to watch your partner masturbate. If they feel shy about demonstrating their technique, they could try using a blindfold. Bear in mind that you'll probably need to be a bit slower/softer than they are with themselves, but their approach will reveal a lot about the speed and strength of grip they prefer.

* **Get into a good position:** Sometimes it's all about having your body in a position that allows you to touch and stimulate so you can get the right rhythm, speed and pressure. Don't endure pain or discomfort; sex injuries are never fun.

* **Adapt to their anatomy:** Try to move your hands with the penis, whether that's moving with the shape, curve or skin. For those who are uncircumcised, you can move the foreskin gently with the motion of your hand, but note that it may be too intense to fully pull the foreskin back and expose the head of the penis. If they are circumcised, the glans may be slightly less sensitive, so try using more lube and playing with the amount of pressure or stimulation.

* **Get with the motions:** Try to keep your motion fluid rather than jerking up and down. Wrap your hand around the penis with about the same amount of pressure you'd use to hold a glass of water, and start by slowly running it up and down. Follow the shape and angle of the penis; most penises will not stand at a perfectly erect 90 degrees. Without removing your hand from the shaft, loosen your grip as you move towards the base of the penis, and move your fingers closer together as you reach the glans of the penis.

* **Mix it up:** Vary your technique. You've got some of the basics, now go and explore. You could try using two hands in a cycle of smooth upstrokes; one hand moves up from the base just as the other reaches the head, or try gently twisting your hand back and forth as you slide it up and down, kinda like a salt and pepper grinder (note, this isn't for everyone!). Explore rubbing your thumb or the palm of your hand in small circles over the tip or frenulum.

* **Blended touch:** Touch other parts of their body – try cupping the testicles, massaging the perineum, or stroking the insides of their thighs.

YOU CAN HAVE A LOT OF FUN WITH A SOFT COCK

Someone yelled this across the room in a workshop once, and it's a reclamation of pleasure that has never left my mind. Penises aren't hard all the time. That's normal. Many people love having a flaccid penis in their mouth or hands. We need to decentre the idea that if a penis isn't hard, you can't have sex. Struggling with erection doesn't necessarily mean that someone isn't attracted to you or that they don't want to have sex with you – there could be a range of other reasons. Don't take their arousal personally, and certainly don't guilt or shame them if they're not performing to your standard. If you or they are struggling, it's always best to seek professional support. See Chapter 6 for more information.

Positions

There are so many positions you can get your body into! And while you may have a favourite go-to, it's likely this will change person to person and experience to experience. It's also worth noting that while I can suggest a few great positions, the best, most mind-blowing sex isn't about what you can contort your body into – it's about attuning to each other, to your needs and desires.

This attunement can be done in a few ways:

※ Checking in and asking questions like, 'What would make this even better?'

※ Syncing your breath cycles to one another, or simply lengthening your breath.

※ Making eye contact.

※ Slowing it right down – you can always add pace.

※ Introducing other sensations you want to experience. Can you add in a cock ring, blindfold, ice cubes …?

Here are some common positions. For illustration reference, refer to pages 170–172.

※ **69 or double mouth to genital:** This is the act of both receiving and giving oral at the same time. Some people love this, while others find it distracting.

✳ **Missionary:** One person lying on their back, the other penetrating.

✳ **Doggy:** Someone on all fours while the other penetrates.

✳ **Spooning:** Big spoon penetrating little spoon.

✳ **Standing:** One or more people standing; the other may be on their back on the bed or bent over, leaning on the bed.

Penis-on-penis sex

Penis-on-penis sex is often called 'gay sex', and unfortunately tends to be treated like something that doesn't require a lot of thought, teaching or nuance. Let's change that. People are having penis-on-penis sex. They always have. If anything, they're having it more than ever, and I hope more people get to experience this too. Our current schooling system and culture has really let down a lot of LGBTQIA+ people. In fact, in 2022, NORMAL surveyed a representative sample of over 1000 Australians and found that most Australian adults received an extremely limited sex education, with only 3 per cent having learnt about safe LGBTQIA+ sex in school.

I have clients who will tell me that penis-on-penis sex wasn't something they experienced for years (even if they really wanted to) because of anxiety and fear. People will say that it's shameful, dangerous, risky or a 'bad thing'. That couldn't be further from the truth.

Common misconceptions

There are a lot of misconceptions about penis-on-penis sex due to homophobia, a lack of sex ed, and limited access to sex-positive information. For so long, sex ed has ignored queer experiences, because of the fear it will corrupt the children!?!!! And seriously, fuck that. It's really important to dispel some of these myths so we can be more open to a range of human experiences.

Myth: There's always a top and always a bottom

Truth: This is true for some but not for all.

Myth: Penis-on-penis sex means you're gay

Truth: Many people enjoy penis-on-penis sex: gay, bi, hetero, pan and a range of genders who may have a penis but don't identify as men: trans, non-binary, genderfluid, etc.

Myth: Penis-on-penis only involves anal penetration

Truth: Anal penetration is one way to have sex, but it's not the only way. Sex means different things for different people.

Myth: Anal penetration should be expected to hurt

Truth: Sex should never involve any unwanted pain.

MUTUAL MASTURBATION

Mutual masturbation is when you masturbate at the same time as someone else. This practice doesn't get the cred it deserves. Mutual masturbation is fairly safe, can help you master your moves better than any sex ed and is a pretty solid way to ensure everyone gets what they want. It can also turn you on, build arousal, and be incorporated as the first stages of foreplay.

Here are a few things to consider:

✳ Are you both masturbating, or is it just one of you?

✳ Do you touch each other at the same time, if you touch each other at all?

✳ Is it a practice or play session? Practice is a time to learn, explore and be clunky, not necessarily orgasmic; while a play session is when we want to put all the skills into real-time and follow the pleasure.

✳ Where and how will you do it? On the bed? Next to each other? On the other side of the room?

Bringing mutual masturbation into your sexual experience can introduce a whole range of benefits to your intimate relationships, sex life and pleasure. If everyone is keen, here are a few techniques you could try:

✳ **Side to side:** You can lie or sit side by side, bodies touching (or not). This position allows you to choose whether you'd like to look at each other. Eye contact can make the experience more intimate.

✳ **Mutual missionary:** Lying on your back with the other on top, either straddling or kneeling between your legs while you touch yourself.

✳ **Full frontal:** Sit facing each other with legs spread (or however you choose) for a full-frontal view of each other.

✳ **Witnessing or being witnessed:** You don't have to masturbate at the same time. Instead, you can decide who will be witnessing and who will be witnessed as they masturbate.

IMPORTANT STUFF

✳ The best technique or touch you can give to someone is one they want to receive, so if you're not sure what to do just ask them.

✳ Everybody is different and your wants and needs can change every time you have sex. In this chapter I've offered dozens of things to try. Explore what feels good for you but be non-attached to the outcome. Don't be surprised if something feels mind-blowing one time and just okay the next.

✳ Create the context for a great time. There is a lot you can do to set the tone and create a safe and sensual environment for everyone involved. And yes, this does involve having a toolkit of sex essentials: lubes, barrier methods, toys, sensory items.

✳ Examine and challenge sexual scripts you've learnt along the way. Most of us have grown up in a homophobic society; it's up to us to change this so all people feel safe and respected in sex and relationships.

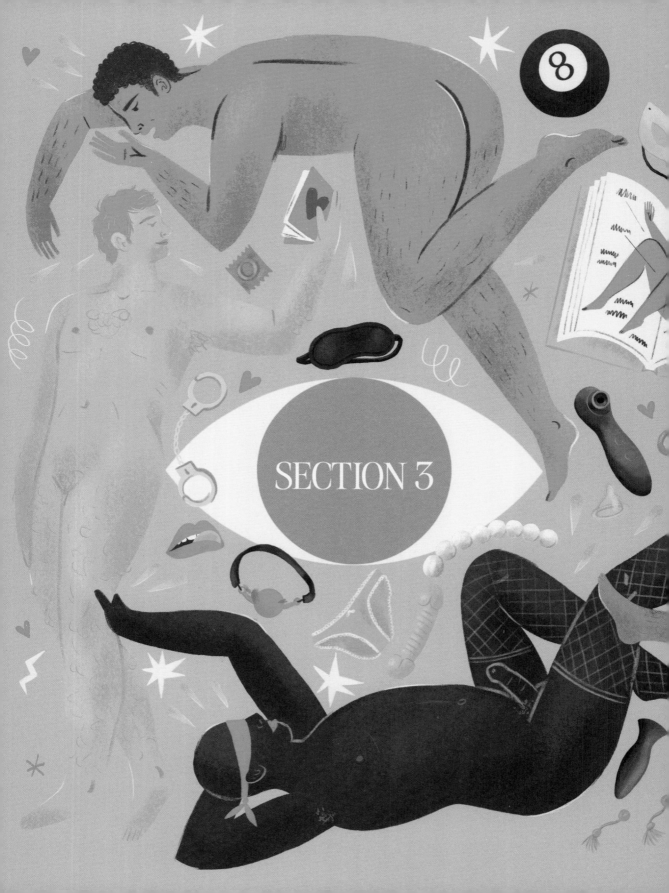

SECTION 3

EXPLORING
PLEASURE

NON-MONOGAMY

What is non-monogamy (NM)? Who is it for and how do we navigate it? This chapter covers the spectrum of relationship dynamics that fall under the NM umbrella, offering a guide to how to have the very first conversation, how to explore ethically and consensually and, of course, the big kicker: navigating jealousy.

In recent years I've noticed a significant increase in people becoming curious about exploring non-monogamy. Their curiosity is often paired with a lot of fear and judgement about what it might mean, the potential thrills and the risks to the foundations of a relationship. Whether you're just curious or you're ready to explore, let's break it down a little further. Non-monogamy is actually a big, ongoing process, and rarely something that just happens.

WHAT IS NON-MONOGAMY?

At the most basic level, non-monogamy is an umbrella term for any relationship that doesn't just feature two people. But this can mean so many things to different people. These relationships may be sexual or romantic, and can be practised by anyone, regardless of their identity or orientation. You may also hear the terms ethical non-monogamy (ENM) or consensual non-monogamy (CNM), which emphasise that the relationship is practised ethically, with honesty, consideration and respect for everyone involved. It's worth noting that a lot of people in non-monogamous structures choose not to include the term 'ethical', because this should be a given. Just because you're not monogamous doesn't mean you're inherently unethical. Dropping the E from ENM works to challenge the idea that the only moral way to have sex, date or be in a relationship is to adopt a monogamous structure.

Some people experience non-monogamy as an inherent part of their identity, just as some experience their queer or straight identity – it can be an integral part of who they are. But for others it's more of a lifestyle, which can feel more like a deliberate or conscious choice to engage in multiple relationships. It may not be an inherent part of someone, but rather a decision they make based on their values, beliefs or preferences. They may adopt a non-monogamous lifestyle because they find it more fulfilling, liberating or aligned with their relationship goals and desires. It can also coexist as both an identity and a lifestyle. Like anything that challenges the normative or linear way of living, practising non-monogamy means you have to constantly deal with judgements, questions and misconceptions.

WHERE TO START?

If you're curious about changing your current relationship structure, know that this doesn't generally happen overnight. I've worked with many couples over months who booked in to open their relationship but may never actually do so. Sometimes they decide it's a one-off thing, like attending a sex party or having a threesome. Others realise that it's an important part of their identity and lifestyle.

For the most part, non-monogamy requires time to process, discuss and set agreements – it's rarely as simple as deciding you'd like to open your relationship and then going all-out.

Non-monogamy can still present unique challenges, even for those who recognise it aligns with their values and the way they want to live and love. For example, I worked with a couple who were both rationally 'cool' with non-monogamy, but who were experiencing a lot of intense emotions in their bodies whenever their partner would go on a date with someone else. They knew they had to keep speaking about it, so when big emotions emerged they started to experiment with the power of a pause: they'd recognise their embodied response and request a pause in the conversation. They'd either take a breath, have five minutes alone to self-regulate or go on a walk and come home at an agreed time. This pause gave them the opportunity to notice what they were feeling and reflect on how their body was responding so they could more effectively communicate a need. They built trust in their own bodies and each other by tuning in to their embodied response. Feeling into it gave them a new way into conversation when they couldn't think their way out of it.

COMMON MISCONCEPTIONS

Myth: You're selfish if you're into non-monogamy

Truth: Selfishness is perceived negatively by society, as it often goes against the values of selflessness and cooperation we value so deeply. But the non-monogamous people in my life are those from whom I've learnt the most about communication, care, respect and autonomy. They view their sexual and romantic partner as an autonomous being with wants and needs of their own, and recognise that they may be their partner but they are not their property. And while it may be challenging to hear about their partner going on a really exciting first date, they can decentre their own experience and be supportive of their partner.

Of course, many people mess up along the way, and it can take time to learn how to practise NM in a way that is kind and aware. But this myth around being selfish is one we need to question. Is it that they are centring their own needs above everyone else's, doing only what they want and not thinking about how their actions affect others? Or is it that they can advocate for their needs, set boundaries and recognise that monogamy is not ideal for them?

Myth: Non-monogamy is just an excuse for cheating

Truth: NM is the opposite, really. It's based on the foundation of honest and consensual agreements with everyone involved. 'Cheating' is breaking boundaries and agreements within a relationship, whereas the foundations of non-monogamy emphasise open communication and ethical behaviour. You can still cheat in non-monogamous relationships by breaking an agreement, and it can feel just as painful. Sex outside of a monogamous agreement is so common, most people have a very personal experience with it. Non-monogamous

people, on the other hand, are able to recognise needs and desires. Instead of breaking an agreement, they create a new structure that works for them.

Myth: People who are non-monogamous are just slutty

Truth: Some NM folk embrace the slut label with open arms as a reclamation of the whorephobic term. They may choose to be non-monogamous because they want to be 'slutty' and have lots of sex with lots of people. But non-monogamy is not solely about sex. People can also be non-monogamous for emotional connections and committed partnerships. It can be about sex, emotions, play or commitment.

Myth: You'll get jealous and break up

Truth: Like any relationship structure, non-monogamy requires ongoing communication, trust and openness to navigate potential challenges. Jealousy can come up, and it often does, just like it may in monogamous relationships. Because it may come up more frequently in non-monogamous relationships, individuals often develop strategies to address and manage jealousy through open dialogue, personal growth and establishing clear boundaries.

Myth: Non-monogamy is a phase or a result of dissatisfaction in a relationship

Truth: Non-monogamy isn't always a response to relationship dissatisfaction; it can be a genuine orientation or a conscious decision to explore different relationship structures that align with personal values and desires. In fact, practitioners will often advise that non-monogamy should not be a band-aid to fix a problem. Instead, you should work on the issues and then introduce it when you're feeling reset, safe and connected.

FEEL INTO WHAT STRUCTURE WORKS FOR YOU!

There's no one-size-fits-all for non-monogamy; there are so many ways to practise with different agreements and structures. While having these labels and structures can be useful, some people may draw inspo and co-create new structures that work for them. Consider the following top-line descriptions as fluid, and not prescriptive.

* **Monogamish:** This is a term coined by author, podcaster and activist Dan Savage to describe a mostly monogamous relationship that allows for other relationships on occasion.

* **Polyfidelity:** More than two people in a closed relationship in which everyone is a primary/equal partner. Typically, all partners are exclusive and are not to be sexually or romantically involved with anyone outside the relationship.

* **Open:** A committed relationship/couple where one or both partners open up to sexual or romantic relationships with others.

* **Swinging:** A couple who has sex with others outside of their relationship. Typically, this is a sexual agreement and they refrain from romantic relationships. This may take place with other people's partners or at parties.

* **Polyamorous:** Poly means many, amor means love – polyamory is the practice of or desire for multiple romantic/sexual relationships with the consent of all people involved.

* **Poly-intimates:** A sexually exclusive couple where each partner has other important emotional, intimate or platonic partnerships.

* **Hierarchical polyamory:** A polyamorous relationship where there is a sense of prioritising one partner (primary) over others (secondary/tertiary).

✳ **Non-hierarchical polyamory:**
A polyamorous relationship structure
where all partners are equal; i.e. there are
no primary partnerships and no hierarchy.

✳ **Solo polyamory:** A person who has
a number of meaningful relationships
without a primary partner.

✳ **Relationship anarchy:** Those who reject
rules associated with conventional
partnership and set their own expectations
and boundaries for relationships. There
is no hierarchy. The philosophy of
relationship anarchy also challenges the
idea that romantic relationships are more
important than all other relationships.

THE NEWLYWEDS

Nicole and Matt, a conservative and
religious couple, were equal parts
curious and concerned about exploring
non-monogamy. Matt proposed it, but he
was concerned about how it would align
with their religious values, whether it was
against their beliefs, and the enduring
feelings of guilt or shame.

Nicole felt insecure about it. She was
worried that Matt's idea of multiple sexual
partners would rock the foundation of
their partnership or create an imbalance
in their emotional connection.

We worked together over a few years
to create safety and establish solid
communication skills. They identified
what felt exciting for both of them and
even attended a sex party and felt
alive and turned on, but realised they
weren't keen to go back. They created
their own relationship structure and
agreement, which was to be open to
future connections but to not actively
seek them. To be free to flirt or go for
a drink, but to check in before anything
sexual happened. They weren't actively
non-monogamous, but they had redefined
their relational agreement. They felt
liberated and free in the dynamic they
created for themselves.

WHAT HAPPENS IF I GET JEALOUS?

People in non-monogamous relationships can still feel jealous, even if it's an active and enthusiastic choice made by everyone involved. My clients will often feel like they're not good at being open when they feel jealous. But feeling jealous doesn't mean you're 'bad', it means you're a human who's experiencing emotions. It can be useful to face the feelings and enquire into the root of the response. More often than not, it can come from fear, or a sense that you're missing out. Try to speak from the feeling, i.e. 'I felt unloved when you chose to go on a date with someone else when I wanted to connect with you.' You'll need to communicate directly to ensure your needs are met – no one is a mind reader (though wouldn't it be nice if everyone could anticipate our needs?). You can revisit the relationship agreements at any point to ensure everyone is fulfilled; it's pretty common to oscillate between opening and closing a relationship.

It's worth noting that some people don't actually experience jealousy. This is often referred to as compersion, which loosely refers to experiencing happiness when your partner is connecting romantically or sexually with another person. A great analogy for this is when your partner gets a promotion, or your best friend goes on a great date. Even though it's not your experience, you're happy for them. Compersion is feeling happy for a partner when they're having fun flirting, dating or having sex with someone else.

WHAT IF IT GOES HORRIBLY WRONG?

As with any romantic relationship, non-monogamy can result in heartbreak if one or more people aren't considerate or aware. Non-monogamy is most fulfilling for all people involved when it is approached willingly and freely, with excitement. If you're uncertain or unsure, it may be worth pausing, or seeking professional support. And if you try it and you're not into it, you can always close your relationship again.

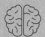 ## Your non-monogamy checklist

No two relationships are the same, and non-monogamy isn't for everyone. It's important to do your research and some honest enquiry before embarking on a new relationship dynamic.

1. **Start with self enquiry:** This is all about understanding your motivations. Take some time to reflect on why you are interested in non-monogamy. It could be a desire for emotional connection with multiple people, exploring diverse relationship dynamics, or aligning with your personal values. Knowing your motivations will help you navigate the journey with clarity. I recommend Jessica Fern's book *Polysecure* as a great place to start. Learn more about the different relationship dynamics that might work for you. Feel into what is most exciting and safe.

2. **Talk about it:** Most people in successful non-monogamous relationships have one thing in common: they talk constantly. Strap in and expect extensive, open, honest and ongoing conversations. Many couples also practise non-violent communication, which focuses on having respect for each other, communicating from a space of care, intending to do no harm and being considerate of intentions and motivations. Check-ins allow you to ensure everyone is happy and comfortable, and to slow things down if needed.

3. **Discuss your boundaries and agreements:** Set clear boundaries that respect the needs and emotions of all parties involved. These boundaries can include agreements on sexual activities, emotional involvement, time management, disclosure of other partners, and so on. A boundary is something you set in relation to others, for example, 'I don't want to hear the intricate details of your dates', and an agreement is something you co-create together, for example, 'We agree to check in after dates'. It can be tempting to set rules like *don't have sex with anyone more than twice*, and while this may create a sense of safety and control, it falls into the territory of monogamous relationships, which have firm rules to not have sex with others. This is why many non-monogamous relationships often opt for boundaries and agreements rather than hard and fast rules.

4. **Schedule ongoing check-ins:** Non-monogamy thrives on open communication. Discuss your desires, boundaries and expectations with your partner(s) or potential partner(s). Regular check-ins are crucial to ensure everyone involved feels heard, respected and comfortable. Acknowledge that jealousy may arise, and learn healthy coping mechanisms to manage it. Openly discussing insecurities and fears can strengthen your relationships. Remember, boundaries may evolve over time, so ongoing communication is essential.

5. **Prioritise safer-sex practices:** Ensure you and your partners practise safer sex and prioritise regular testing for STIs. You'll need to discuss how you and your partner(s) want to navigate this. Consistent and open communication about sexual health is vital to maintain a safe and responsible non-monogamous lifestyle.

6. **Make time for ongoing self-reflection:** Regularly reflect on your own feelings, motivations and personal growth. Non-monogamy can be a transformative experience that challenges societal norms and encourages personal development. Set regular check-ins for yourself.

7. **Consider others:** Partner privilege refers to the advantages or benefits that can come from being in a committed or intimate relationship with someone. It acknowledges that having a partner can provide certain advantages, such as emotional support, companionship, shared responsibilities and access to resources. For those who have a primary partner or are opening up their relationship, it's important to recognise and appreciate partner privilege while also being mindful of the responsibilities to maintain a healthy and equitable relationship with others. It's really common for a 'third' or secondary partner to feel unseen, unheard or undervalued. I've had many in my practice room saying that they've felt used. Even if someone isn't your primary partner, everyone involved deserves to be treated with care and respect.

8. **Seek support:** Join non-monogamy communities, attend workshops or seek therapy for insights, advice and support.

IMPORTANT STUFF

✳ More people are getting curious about non-monogamy.

✳ At the most basic level, non-monogamy is an umbrella term for any relationship that doesn't just feature two people. This can mean many things to different people.

✳ Some people experience non-monogamy as an inherent part of their identity, just as some experience their queer or straight identity – it can be an integral part of who they are. But for others it's more of a lifestyle, and can feel more like a deliberate or conscious choice to engage in multiple relationships.

✳ There are so many ways to practise with different agreements and structures. While having these labels and structures can be useful for some, others may co-create new structures that work for them.

✳ People in non-monogamous relationships can still feel jealous, even if non-monogamy is an active and enthusiastic choice made by everyone involved.

✳ You can open and close your relationship as you wish.

✳ Non-monogamy is not for everyone, just like monogamy isn't for everyone. But many couples feel more aligned, connected and excited by their non-monogamous relationships, and wouldn't want it any other way.

TOYS

Can I get addicted to my vibe? Does needing toys make me a bad lover? What if it feels unnatural? Sex toys have one function: to make sex feel good. There's a whole lot of shame, stigma and misinformation that may affect our experience with using them, but I have seen and heard infinite stories of toys transforming sex for many. Sex toys are useful, normal and, for some people, essential.

A friend bought me one of my first sex toys. It was a powerful magic wand but to use it I had to plug it into the wall. Depressingly, the cord was too short, and the only power point in my bedroom was two metres away from my bed, near my door, which meant I had to squat near the wall. This really added to the sense of impending dread that my housemates would hear the powerful motor or accidentally walk in.

Sex toys have come a long way. With the majority of new toys coming with USB chargers and quiet motors, no member of the younger generation will ever have to worry about cord length or housemates hearing them maz. Not only have the functions and experience improved, but aesthetically they've also moved well beyond the glittery, jelly, veiny-phallic dildos of the early 2000s. Over the past few years we've seen toys emerge that look like something you'd keep on your bedside table, rather than hidden within it. They are easy to use, safe, and their only function is to make sex feel great.

At the start of my career I learnt how important toys are for sex. Personally, I was on board. I'd had a really exciting and positive experience with toys (before and after the magic-wand era), but in working and studying with a diverse group of people, I learnt how essential toys are in allowing more bodies to access pleasure. I discovered the positive impact vibrator use can have on sexual arousal and function , and I saw how toys were considered 'nice to have' for some, while for others toys were a reliable and important tool in all sexual experiences and could also validate their gender identity and expression. Toys help

people to feel pleasure. They've enabled many of my clients to experience orgasm for the first time and are especially useful for people with vulvas who have a lot of penetrative sex with limited clit stimulation, allowing them to climax as often as their cis male counterparts. Toys encourage us to move beyond the heteronormative ideal that sex is only about genitals banging up against each other.

In 2020, Lucy Wark and I launched NORMAL, a sexual wellness company that makes toys and lubes and provides free sex ed. Over the years we have done research into human sexuality, conducted smaller surveys of our community and discovered the challenges people face in buying sex toys. For some, the barrier is not knowing where to start; for others, it's shame and fear; and for others, it can feel daunting to invest in a toy without knowing whether they'll even like it. Sex ed is often crucial in supporting people to find the right toy and then learn how to use it. NORMAL has now created an extensive library on how to choose, use and integrate toys into all sexual experiences. For more information, I've included a QR code at the end of this chapter that will lead you to free resources.

COMMON MISCONCEPTIONS

Myth: You're not a good sexual partner if you need toys

Truth: Being open to toys or supporting someone's use of sex toys actually makes you a great sexual partner. It shows them that you've deconstructed the idea that sex is about a performance, and that you value their pleasure. Using toys on your own or with a partner doesn't mean you're having problems in the bedroom or that you're boring. It shows that you're comfortable, curious and prioritise feeling good.

Myth: Sex toys will ruin partnered sex

Truth: This one comes back to the old-school patriarchal belief that sex should be between *a man and a woman who love each other deeply*, and that all sexual choices must be made to benefit the relationship. It is dangerous to suggest someone needs to 'save' their body for partnered sex, and that masturbation will ruin future 'lovemaking'. Everyone is entitled to experience pleasure in a way that feels fulfilling. Using toys solo can be a great learning tool to make partnered sex even better. I'm not suggesting that you should only masturbate with the goal of enhancing partnered sex; rather, I'm hoping to dispel the myth that it'll ruin you for partnered sex. It will actually make you a better lover. The more you learn about your body, the easier it is to communicate your needs to a partner and integrate this knowledge into sex.

Myth: Toys will damage your nerve endings

Truth: You can't rub away nerve endings! They don't work like that. Think about it this way: if I put a vibrator on my arm for five minutes a day, I'm not going to vibrate away the sensation in my arm. If anything, I'm bringing more awareness to my arm, strengthening neural pathways. The *Journal of Sexual Medicine* found that a majority of people don't experience any genital symptoms associated with vibrator use. It is non-medical and fearmongering to suggest that vibrators will damage you – this idea is more about shaming people (particularly people with vulvas) for masturbating. There is no evidence to suggest sex toys desensitise you.

UNTOUCHED

A client of mine bought a sex toy in an impulsive moment of sexual curiosity. But by the time it arrived, the shame and fear had settled in. She put the sealed, unopened box in her top drawer and ignored it. She booked in to see me after she gave birth to her first baby, as she'd never had an orgasm. Over a few months we covered all the bases: sex education and anatomy, building awareness in her body, masturbation techniques, practices to try with her husband. But she wasn't feeling anything. When she told me that she wanted to try her toy but was overwhelmed by not knowing how to use it, and the subsequent shame that came from both wanting and not knowing, I thought we needed a safe entry point of exposure. I asked if she'd feel comfortable bringing it to the session, and she did.

In the room, she unwrapped it and held it in her hand, noting how soft it felt, and how much she liked the colour and shape. I then invited her to turn it on and go through the different vibration modes. I guided her through a practice of awakening sensation in her hands using the vibe, in which she learnt how to follow pleasure to the areas of the hand that felt best – without the pressure of trying to make her hand cum. She noted how nice and how safe it felt. Her homework was to take that practice of awakening sensation, free from goal, and bring it to a non-genital erogenous zone first (i.e. neck, chest, nipples) and then after that to bring the vibration to her genitals and similarly follow the pleasure.

By the next session, she'd had her first ever orgasm. The toy was the final tool she needed to help her climax. She had done a lot of work prior in unpacking and reframing sexual shame, as well as ongoing masturbation practices and learning foundational somatic tools. But it was the toy that got her there. And not only did she learn to climax with a toy, but because she had learnt what her body needed through the toy, over the next few weeks she learnt how to climax without a vibrator. Her vibrator didn't ruin her, it helped her.

Some people may start to feel 'numb' after extended use of a toy in one session, just like they may feel overly sensitive after receiving oral, or penetration, for a long period. They may also feel reliant on their toys to climax and want to start exploring new ways to cum.

The antidote to all of this is to switch up the masturbation routine. Try using a different hand or alternating between using hands only in one session then vibration in the next, or by bringing more of your body into the experience, like your breath, movement, sound, touch and placement of awareness. Try pausing and doing things differently. The sensation always returns; you can always find new ways to access pleasure.

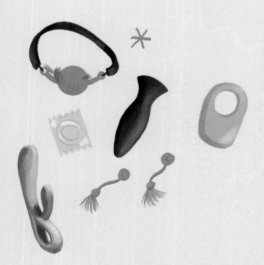

TYPES OF TOYS

✳ **Vibrators**: Consider this an umbrella term for any toy that vibrates.

✳ **Clit suction or air pulse**: These toys have completely revolutionised pleasure for people with clits, introducing many to their first orgasm. These innovative toys use suction and/or air pulsation to create a gentle or intense sucking sensation on the clitoris. They can provide unique, indirect stimulation and are often designed to feel like the best oral you'll ever have.

✳ **Bullet**: These small, discreet vibrators look like a bullet, or sometimes a lipstick. They're versatile, and can be used to stimulate various erogenous zones, including the clitoris, nipples or even the perineum. They're great for targeted pleasure, and can be easily incorporated into solo or partnered play.

✳ **G-spot vibrator or dildo**: Specifically designed to stimulate the G-spot, these generally have a curved or bulbous shape to target the G-spot directly.

✳ **Magic wand:** These powerful larger external vibrators not only look like a wand but fittingly live up to their name, thanks to the many orgasms they've granted over the decades. Originally manufactured as a back massager, they are now most well known and loved as a vibrator. They usually have a flexible head that can be used for external stimulation on any part of the body.

✳ **Cock rings:** Cock rings are worn around the base of the penis or the base of the penis and testicles. They can help enhance and maintain erections by restricting blood flow, creating a pleasurable experience for both partners. Some are flexible and made out of silicone and rubber, while others are hard and made out of metals. If you're new to cock rings, I recommend starting with a soft material and always, always using lube – and plenty of it! Put the ring on when you're not erect, or only semi-erect – it may be uncomfortable or painful otherwise. As you're restricting blood flow, make sure you only leave it on for a maximum of 20 to 30 minutes.

✳ **Dildos:** These toys are used for penetration and thrusting to access pleasure points deeper in the body. They can be made of various materials, such as silicone, glass or metal, and come in different sizes, textures and colours. Often dildos have a solid structure and form to manually stimulate the prostate, G-spot, A-spot or other pleasurable areas.

✳ **Penis sleeve:** Sleeves are mostly designed for penises, and can be used in both solo and partnered sex, to up-level hand jobs and blow jobs. Basically, with the soft material and texture, they make everything feel more intense; the lube often stays in the sleeve, meaning you don't need to reapply, and some even have a vibration mode that can stimulate sensitive areas like the frenulum. Sleeves can make hand jobs, blow jobs and masturbation feel more intense and pleasurable, but I also often recommend a sleeve to clients who are learning to delay ejaculation in partnered sex so they can practise building and down-regulating arousal with a tool that creates more sensation than their hand.

✳ **Fleshlight:** They look like flashlights and they come in a range of skin colours and tones, designed for penises to simulate the feeling of penetration. They unfortunately have a bad rap because they often look poorly made or like rubber genitals (which is certainly a thing for some, but for many it can be off-putting). They're typically soft, flexible, and textured to feel like either a vagina or anus. Some even have a silicon anus or vulva on the top part.

✳ **Kegel balls:** Kegel balls are designed to strengthen the pelvic floor muscles. They can be inserted into the vagina and provide stimulation, with some offering a vibration mode while providing a workout for those muscles.

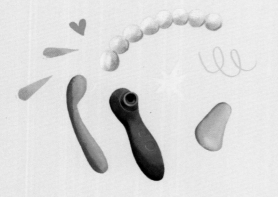

✳ **BDSM toys:** The options are endless. Some of the more common examples include handcuffs, blindfolds, paddles and bondage restraints. I recommend learning from a professional if you want to engage in pain play, to ensure you are practising as safely as possible – see Chapter 15 for more on this.

✳ **Butt plugs:** A butt plug is a sex toy with a flared base and a more cylindrical head. This can feel good for those who like anal, blended stimulation, prostate play or more intense orgasms. They can be used solo or during partnered sex.

✳ **Prostate massagers:** Designed to massage the prostate, these toys are curved up to stimulate the anterior (front side) of the body, where the prostate is. They will also have a flared base, which is great for perineum stimulation.

✳ **Anal beads:** They look like a string of beads. People like to use these when they enjoy the feeling of something being progressively pulled out or inserted at the peak of orgasm. The beads can come in a range of shapes and sizes.

✳ **Double-ended dildos**: They feature a dildo on both ends, allowing both partners to experience penetration simultaneously.

✳ **Strap-ons**: Typically consisting of a harness that holds a dildo, strap-ons come in a variety of sizes, shapes and materials to suit different preferences. There are also underwear strap-ons, which are like your classic undies just with a hole for the dildo, and vibrating strap-ons with a built-in vibrator in the dildo, which can enhance pleasure for both the wearer and their partner. Strapless strap-ons are typically double-ended and allow for a hands-free experience for the wearer. They are inserted into the vagina or anus, allowing the wearer to penetrate their partner while also being penetrated, without the need for a harness. Hollow strap-ons are designed for people with erectile difficulties or those looking to add extra length or girth. They can be worn by individuals with a penis, allowing them to maintain an erection during penetration.

ANAL TOYS

There's an anal toy for every bum, and people choose specific features that work for them. It's important, though, to take note of the following things:

✳ All anal toys *must* have a flared base. Do not push past the flared base.

✳ Use plenty of lube.

✳ Thoroughly clean toys after use, especially if you plan on putting it in a vagina or anywhere else.

✳ Don't push through any unwanted pain.

✳ Bigger is not always better – work your way up.

QUESTIONS TO ASK WHEN SHOPPING FOR TOYS

If you're keen to explore, ask yourself the following questions to help you choose the right toy(s) for you:

* What sexual experiences do you want to use it for?

* What do you like the look of?

* What body part(s) do you want to stimulate?

* Who is it for?

* What are your boundaries?

* What are your sexual needs? Quiet motor? Waterproof?

HOW TO USE SEX TOYS WITH A PARTNER

When you use sex toys with a partner, there are a few things you want to cover to make sure you're both comfortable. But first, talk about it. (Refer to Chapter 8, where I've included a guide on how to talk about sex.) Talk about the benefits, dispel any myths, answer their questions, then go shopping together to find something that's exciting for everyone.

I recommend trying it solo first to learn about the toy and how you'd like to use it on yourself. Then doing a show and tell–style session to teach your partner all about what you like. This is where a practice-and-play approach might come in handy. Set aside 15 to 30 minutes to practise, check in constantly, and try not to be attached to the outcome. This is your opportunity to learn; you don't need to be experts straight away. Then set aside another 15 to 30 minutes for your play session. Again, it isn't orgasm-focused; rather, you're just putting into action all the things you learnt in your practice session.

Trying something new can feel daunting. If you need more information or ideas on how to approach this, follow this QR code to the NORMAL website for dozens of explainers, videos and tools to explore when you're using toys with partners.

How to incorporate different toys

The options are pretty endless here. Some people use toys to build arousal, others add them to penetrative sex, and others may be more into mutual masturbation. It's often easier, if you're the one receiving the stimulation, to hold the toy, as you know what your body needs, and it can be a bit hit or miss. But you could also ask your partner to use it on your nipples, vulva or perineum or to provide anal stimulation. You can also use it to bring your partner close to orgasm with vibration before pulling back multiple times to build to a more intense peak (a technique known as edging).

Many toys you use solo can also be integrated into outercourse, self-stimulation, edging, mutual masturbation and adding extra stimulation to a penetrative position (e.g. clitoral stimulation during vaginal or anal sex).

Whenever you're using toys:

- ✳ Build arousal in the whole body before going straight to the genitals – it'll make it feel so much better.

- ✳ Lube up your toys – it'll help it glide across or into all sensitive areas.

- ✳ Continue with all other sexual play to increase blended sensation.

- ✳ Move your body – sure, you could just get the toy in place and let it do its thing, but it'll feel so much better if you move your hips, touch other body parts or kiss while using it.

- ✳ Explore different positions, such as mutual masturbation, lying on your back, sitting up facing each other or being penetrated from behind while using toys.

If at any point it hurts, is uncomfortable or no longer feels like a great idea, stop and check in. Do not endure unwanted pain – toys should only be about giving pleasure. For more info on how to use toys, use the QR code on the previous page.

IMPORTANT STUFF

✳ Sex toys can help you have the best sex of your life.

✳ Toys are certainly not for everyone, so if you're
not into them – cool! Go you.

✳ If you or a sexual partner is interested, do your research,
talk about it, find something that turns you on and explore
ways to integrate it into solo or partnered sex.

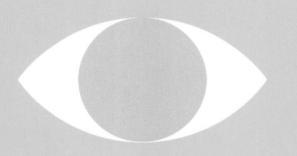

KINK, FETISH AND BDSM

Is it weird that I'm into 'that'? What's the difference between a kink and a fetish? How will I know if I'm into it? How do I keep myself and my partners safe? BDSM has become more mainstream in recent years, but there's a lot you have to learn before exploring it. In this chapter we'll look at the basics of kink, aka anything that bends from the straight and narrow.

Pop culture, porn and media have accelerated our collective intrigue and fascination with kink, fetish and BDSM. This topic elicits a pretty visceral response in many. For some it's excitement and arousal; for others it's disgust and fear. Whether you're interested in exploring it yourself or you just want to learn more, this curiosity is common, though how you actually go about it will be different for everyone. Kink, fetish and BDSM don't have to involve pain, power dynamics or dressing head to toe in latex – though they certainly can.

This topic rightly belongs in the exploration section of this book, as it really should be considered advanced play. I say this with no judgement, but rather with the considered awareness of someone who has practised, studied and played with many elements throughout my professional and personal life. Much of this book has been inspired by my learnings of being in kinky spaces, where I was able to refine how I understood consent, communication, playfulness, queerness, foreplay, arousal, aftercare, creativity, attunement and pleasure as a tool for healing. When BDSM is practised well and by people who know what they're doing, it can change the way we experience sex and our bodies. It can be transformative.

However, it is one of the most distressing parts of my job when I hear about someone manipulating the practice of BDSM as a cover for their abuse or assault of a sexual partner. In recent years, I've seen an increase in presentations of cis men choking partners without consent, shaming them for not being into pain play and pressuring them to engage in power dynamics they're not interested in. This is not kink; this is sexual assault.

This chapter is a celebration of kink and sexual exploration. I want to focus on how to do kink really well, so that everyone involved leaves feeling more human.

THE DIFFERENCE BETWEEN A KINK AND A FETISH

A kink is an experience, fantasy or desire that you may find arousing, something that falls outside of the straight-and-narrow definition of sex and sexuality (think of it like a 'kink' in a piece of string). This might be BDSM, spanking, impact play, dirty talk, role play, etc. Kinks are really subjective: what's kinky for some, may not be kinky for others.

A fetish is when someone places high sexual value on an object, body part or activity that may or may not be of a sexual nature. For some people, a fetish must be present for the person to experience arousal and orgasm, but this isn't the case for everyone. The most well-known fetish is foot play (toe-sucking, needing to see their partner's feet, wearing high-heels, etc.), but a fetish can really include anything that is explored as part of sex with full consent from all participants.

You're not alone if at times you find the distinction confusing – there can be an overlap between a kink and a fetish. Think of a kink as something someone likes to have, and a fetish as something someone needs to have.

Kinks and fetishes are often pathologised. Let me be clear: you don't need 'daddy issues' to enjoy them, nor is there anything wrong with having a number of kinks or fetishes. Sure, some people have found that their kinks and fetishes have allowed them to process uncomfortable or traumatic experiences from their past, because they have had safe spaces to feel autonomous, in control and safe. But not everyone explores kinks or fetishes for this reason.

As you read the following list of common kinks and fetishes, I invite you to observe how your body responds. You may realise you're more kinky than you gave yourself credit for, or you may even be a bit disturbed or disgusted by what you read. That's okay; you're human and we all respond in different ways. Perhaps you can opt for curiosity over judgement.

SOME COMMON KINKS AND FETISHES

- ✳ **BDSM:** The abbreviation can be divided into Bondage, Discipline, Dominance, Submission, Sadism, Masochism. This includes a wide range of activities too: power dynamics, control, spanking, blindfolding, dom/sub arrangements and pain play.

- ✳ **Dom/Sub:** A power dynamic or relational agreement where one person takes the role of dom ('dominant', or leading) and the other is sub ('submissive'), often experienced in the context of BDSM.

- ✳ **Spanking:** The impact of a hand or fingers on muscular/fatty parts of the body such as the buttocks or thighs (never over bone or organs).

- ✳ **Voyeurism:** The act of watching other people have sex. Mirror play is great for this one, as are any group sex experiences.

- ✳ **Role play:** Where your pleasure is heightened by playing the 'role' of someone other than yourself, e.g. nurse and patient, librarian and student, alien and astronaut – go off, my friends.

* **Dirty talk:** Verbal communication used to build arousal and/or express needs during, before or after sex. This can include everything from requests (*Slower/Deeper/Touch me here/I want you …*), to descriptions (*You're so bad/ hot/wet/hard, I've been naughty*).

* **Nipple play:** This may surprise you because it's pretty popular, but nipple play is a kink! It's mostly enjoyed via tweaking, licking, sucking or nibbling a partner's nipples, or experiencing sensation in your own nipples.

* **Hosiery:** Lingerie, tights, pantyhose – you or your partner(s) may experience more arousal wearing or seeing hosiery.

* **Auralism:** If the sound of your partner's moan turns you on, you may have a sound kink. Explore yours through ASMR or the sound effects on audio erotica.

* **Praise kink:** When a person finds compliments, words of affirmation or positive feedback arousing/ pleasurable, e.g. *Good girl/boy/ mummy/daddy* or *You're so good at …*

* **Spit:** We've all got it. This kink involves spit play, either dripping or spitting in or on someone.

* **Ropes or bondage:** A well-known kink for those who enjoy the feeling of restricting or being restricted.

* **Blindfolds:** Also known as amaurophilia. This kink involves a preference for sex with sensory deprivation, to explore heightened senses, power dynamics, teasing or for those who enjoy having sex in complete darkness.

* **Orgasm control:** Where one partner controls the timing of the other's orgasm. This can be experienced through edging or bondage.

* **Anilingus:** Any sexual act that stimulates the anus via licking, kissing or other oral stimulation.

* **Food play:** Incorporating food as a sensual experience (think whipped cream, melted chocolate over the body, frozen foods for temperature play or 'sploshing').

* **Melolagnia:** Being turned on by music, a singer's voice, the beat or composition of a song that can lead to physical sensations and arousal.

* **Piss play:** Also known as urophilia – for those with a kink for 'golden showers'.

* **Vicarious arousal:** A kink for hearing the sexual experiences and behaviours of others, also known as vicarphilia, often enjoyed through erotic podcasts and audiobooks.

* **Temperature play:** A different way of enhancing and exploring sensation during sex. Examples include wax play, ice-cold kisses, gently warming your sex toys or lube, and running an ice cube over erogenous zones. Always check that the temp is body safe before playing.

* **Group sex:** Threesomes, orgies (more than three), double penetration, daisy chains (a chain of people giving/receiving oral) and group mutual masturbation are just a few ways a group sex kink can be fulfilled.

* **Exhibitionism:** Behaviours that intend to attract attention.

I want to remind you here that regardless of the sex you're having, it should never involve any *unwanted* pain. As soon as it becomes unwanted, everything needs to stop. If you're keen to explore new things, I recommend attending a workshop, taking a course or seeing a trained professional to learn new skills before diving head-first into it – especially if it involves any sort of pain and anything that could cause long-term harm to the body.

YOUR ADVANCED PLAY CHECKLIST

* Have you researched or learnt about this new thing?

* Have you discussed and set clear boundaries?

* Have you practised communicating outside of a sexual context, and does everyone involved understand what clear consent is?

* Are you prepared to start slow?

* Is there anywhere you don't want to be touched?

* Is there anything you don't want?

* What do you want?

* Where do you want to focus?

* How will you check in afterwards?

* What is your aftercare?

Try to get as much information from your partner as possible, and share, in as much detail as possible, about your own boundaries. The more they know, the better. This is often a really exhilarating part of the process. Following the simple checklist on the previous page is an easy way to make sure this experience is great for everyone. Remember, different people have different levels of comfort, and it's important that everyone is happy to be there, free to leave whenever they want, safe, and enjoying themselves.

SETTING BOUNDARIES

Boundary setting is obviously important for all types of sex, and we've already covered this at length in Chapter 7. I urge you to revisit that chapter and do all the activities I've set before jumping into kink or BDSM. Building on the skills you've practised, there are a few other ways you can choose to give and receive consent that are typical to kink scenes.

Using a safe word or phrase is famously adopted in kinky sex as a way to communicate that you want to stop. Choose a word that you would never ordinarily use in the bedroom, like *pineapple* or *palm tree*, and agree

on it ahead of time so that when it is said, everyone knows to stop immediately and check in.

Another really popular tool is the traffic light system. This works just like a traffic light: saying the word 'green' means go, 'orange' means pause or slow down and 'red' means stop immediately. If you're doing something that means you can't talk then you'll need to come up with hand or head gestures, a sound, or another, more physical form of safe word. If your mouth is covered, compromised or pressed into the pillow, it may not be practical to use a safe word. Decide ahead of time on a physical signal that means 'stop', like two taps on your partner's arm or a poke with your toes.

Choose something that is easy to say and isn't used as part of a role play situation. In some role plays, people may want to play with the words *don't, no* or *stop* as cues to continue the scenario or sexual act. In this case, everyone involved would need to come up with another term, like *lemonade*, or use the traffic light system. Any word can be a safe word, so long as everyone is clear on what it is. Make sure you practise saying it, hearing it and respecting it before engaging in the act.

SPANKING

The first time I was spanked properly was in a workshop and I was paired with Bob, an older gay man. He was slightly confronted and cautious because he'd never touched a woman's bottom before, and in that moment, I'd never felt more safe. In the workshop we were learning about power dynamics and how to spank safely. It wasn't a sexual experience for me and Bob, but in other contexts spanking can build sexual arousal or erotic gratification for the spanker and/or spankee.

It can be a sex act in itself; one person may be lying over another's knees while they are spanked with varying levels of intensity and/or duration. Or spanking may be integrated into sex; one person may be getting spanked while being penetrated. It can also be incorporated into role play and involve other tools like a paddle or wooden spoon. Spanking is also a great introduction into something more kinky if you're new to the pleasure/pain dynamic.

Here's how you might approach spanking for the first time, but these ideas could be loosely applied to exploring anything new.

Start gently

As with anything new, but particularly when exploring impact and pain play, we want to start light and slow, only intensifying at the request of the receiver. Your version of a light touch might be different from someone else's, which is why you should be constantly checking in with your partner(s) about how it feels or how you can make it feel even better. Use the palm of your hand for a louder noise/wider smack, and your fingers for tapping different regions.

Where should you spank?

We want to aim for the more muscular and fatty body parts, like the bum or thighs. While some people love to receive touch around their nipples and chest, it's best to ease into these erogenous zones. Never spank bones or over organs. Spanking the lower half of the buttocks in an upwards direction can gently vibrate and build arousal in the genitals.

Variety and pace

When you spank someone, you're trying to increase blood flow to an area, so when you notice the skin starting to get more pink or red or it starts to feel hot, the skin will be sensitive. Pause regularly throughout to offer variety in sensation like tickling, kissing, blowing cool air or using feathers. This can feel intense and pleasurable, and also gives the person being spanked a break before the impact returns. As an example, you may give a few spanks in the same area then hold, soothe, kiss or ease the sensitive area before building up the intensity again.

Verbal and nonverbal cues

I encourage constant check-ins when it comes to spanking. While verbal feedback is great, look for nonverbal cues too. If their body feels tense, ease it up, check in, pause, stop and/or rework your touch. You may want to bring in the traffic light system here. You could ask: 'Was that a red (stop), orange (pause) or green (go!)?' or you could say something like, 'We'll start light and build intensity' or 'On a scale of 1 to 10, how intense was that?' or 'Can we go harder/faster/softer?'

Brand new to spanking?

As always, if you're hoping to try something new with your partner(s), an open conversation is the way to go. Do your own research about how or where you'd like to be spanked, then make time to chat with them in a context that feels safe, comfortable and outside of the sex zone

(not during, right before or after). If they're keen, great! If they're not, that's cool – let them know you respect their boundaries and thank them for sharing them. You can always incorporate spanking/tapping/impact into your solo play.

DON'T FORGET THE AFTERCARE

This stuff is so important that I've included a whole section on it in Chapter 10. However, I also wanted to pay homage to this particular practice within this chapter, as aftercare was first created and practised in kink communities. If you've just done something particularly intense, both you and your partner might be feeling exhilarated afterwards, or a bit vulnerable too. This is often referred to as 'sub drop' or 'dom drop', describing the emotional drop you might experience afterwards. You can counter these feelings with some aftercare. Debrief with your partner, cuddle, make each other a cup of tea, offer physical or emotional affection. It's pretty shitty behaviour to end sex by immediately rolling over and looking at your phone, but particularly so after an advanced play. Use this time to be intimate with your partner, check in on them, and make sure you're both comfortable and happy with how everything went.

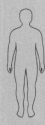

Trying it out

In speaking with my clients, I've noticed that a few acts feel more accessible at the start. Some people didn't even realise that what they were exploring fell under the kink umbrella. Here are some examples:

✳ **Sensation play:** This is a powerful practice that many people love and benefit from. Try exploring sensation play using a blindfold. Explore a range of sensory items like ice cubes, strawberries, something soft like a feather and something firm like a paddle.

✳ **Wax play:** Make sure you only play with a candle that is body safe and made with the purpose of being dripped on bodies; others can cause long-term harm. (Read the instructions on the packet to make sure you're using the sex candles safely.) Start in less sensitive areas. Hold the candle at a distance from the body and start slow. Many people like to include an ice cube and run it across the area.

✳ **Act out a fantasy:** Choose a fantasy you've always wanted to live out and enact it together. Talk about what turns you on and why, and what your hopes are for the fantasy. See if you can identify any BDSM elements that appeal to you within the dynamic – are restraints, dirty talk or impact play involved? Focus on a single element of BDSM and bring it to life in the fantasy you create. Some people may just want to talk it through and that can feel kinky enough. Others may want to put it all into practice.

✳ **Start small:** It's tempting to go all-out and stock up on latex, paddles, restraints and blindfolds. Instead, start by focusing on one small thing and branching out from there. If your partner's into spanking, for example, you don't need to buy an arsenal of whips right away. Start slow and use your hand for spanking, and debrief afterwards together. If they loved it, great – you can go a little harder next time or get a paddle or a flogger. But when you're starting out it's always better to be saying 'That was great, let's do more next time!' than 'That went a bit too far for me.'

IMPORTANT STUFF

✳ A kink is an experience, fantasy or desire that you may find arousing, something that falls outside of the straight-and-narrow definition of sex and sexuality. This could be BDSM, spanking, impact play, dirty talk, role play, etc.

✳ A fetish is when someone places high sexual value on an object, body part or activity that may or may not be of a sexual nature. Some people need a fetish to be present for them to experience arousal and orgasm, but this isn't the case for everyone.

✳ Sex should never involve any *unwanted* pain. As soon as it becomes unwanted, everything stops.

✳ Boundary setting is obviously important for all types of sex, but it's particularly important for those who are into kink. In fact, we can learn some of the best consent and boundary setting practices from kink communities.

✳ Don't yuck anyone's yum. You may not be into it, and that's great that you're aware of your boundary, but it's important to be kind and respectful.

PORN

Am I watching too much porn? Why can
I no longer climax without visual stimulus?
Is there a way to watch porn more ethically?
Attitudes and ideas from porn and pop
culture can shape how we feel about
ourselves and what we expect during sex.
Learn about how to unpack these messages,
find inspiration in erotica and engage with
your cultural influences in a healthy way.

People watch porn for pleasure, exploration, stress relief,
distraction, inspiration, education and boredom. They
watch porn to climax, but they also watch porn when there's
nothing else to do. Whatever it is that drives us to watch
porn, undoubtedly the things we watch, read and listen to
influence the way we experience sex. I see the way porn
affects people.

Porn is a performance, and watching it without acknowledging that each scene is the result of planning meetings, discussion around what will take place in the scene, lunch breaks and hours of editing leads viewers to think they should have sex the way they do in porn. But although many people learn about sex through porn, porn isn't created for educational purposes, it's created as entertainment.

The purpose of porn is to turn you on, stimulate you, arouse your brain and make you climax. It's important to remember this. I'm not going to focus on the porn industry in this chapter (because let's face it, it's fucking huge). Rather, I'll be looking at how we can consume it in a more mindful, ethical and self-regulated way. People will never stop watching porn and as we all know, if you tell someone not to do something, it'll only energise the forbidden.

AM I ADDICTED TO PORN?

Fear of porn addiction comes up a lot in session. Clients will notice that they need porn to climax, or that they have to fantasise about something else in order to build arousal in their body.

A 2016 *Journal of Sexual Medicine* study found that self-perceived porn addiction, in which a person perceives themselves to be addicted to porn, is not a formally recognised disorder, even though it is something that's being talked about a lot. A 2019 study published in the *Journal of Clinical Medicine* also acknowledged that porn addiction is a huge topic, but said it was difficult to pinpoint at what point pornography use became addiction, or at what point it became problematic for an individual.

Addiction is often defined as a chronic dysfunction of the brain system. It is craving a substance or behaviour with little regard for consequence. Addiction involves reward, motivation and memory, and those who are addicted can experience a compulsive or obsessive pursuit of reward. As an extension of this, porn addiction involves feeling like you can't stop watching it, even if it is affecting you negatively and you want to stop. It becomes an addiction when the obsession affects your relationships with your own body or with others, your work or other parts of life. For those who feel they are addicted to or reliant on porn, it will be useful to seek professional support.

While not everyone will become addicted to porn, many will identify that it affects the way they think and feel about sex. Here are a few ways porn can negatively impact people:

✳ **Porn can affect sexual expectations**: This is the big one. Mainstream porn is a performance; often the positions and duration of the act are not possible or pleasurable for most people. Porn is crafted with stimulation in mind. I'll often have clients concerned that they ejaculate prematurely because they can't last for an hour. They don't realise that lasting for ten minutes is completely normal and healthy; instead, they compare themselves to the actors on screen who last for over an hour, without acknowledging that, as on all film sets, the actors have breaks.

✳ **Porn can reinforce sexual scripts**: Porn often depicts mind-blowing, leg-trembling orgasms from penetration alone. Vaginal orgasm is often misrepresented as the 'best' way for cis women to orgasm (read: the easiest for people with penises), but it's often the most difficult for people with vulvas. We know that the majority of people with vulvas will need clitoral stimulation, and that the majority aren't getting enough of it. It's a stock standard porn scene where a person with a vulva receives no foreplay, external stimulation or even lube, and after three seconds of penetrative sex is writhing with pleasure.

✳ **It can create stimulation reliance**: If you're masturbating to the same stimulus, using the same hand, same position, your body starts to anticipate that type of stimulation. This means that when it comes to having sex in a different way, it may be more difficult to become aroused.

✳ **It can lack clear consent and communication**: Unlike healthy sexual experiences, porn often skips the fundamentals. Consent, communication, contraception and protection are rarely represented or explained. In some porn, performers do very little talking and can jump into any new position or sex act at any moment. This in itself isn't a problem – everyone communicates consent in their own way – but when we see people having hardcore explicit or more 'advanced' sex with no discussion of consent at all, it can make us think that that's how sex is meant to be. And it isn't. Before any good porn production begins, the performers will sit down and have a discussion about what they're about to do, offering each other informed consent about the acts that will take place. This is vital to any sexual experience, whether on camera or off. Without consent, sex of any kind simply cannot happen.

✳ **Children can easily access it**: Porn is easily accessible for children and young minds who can't distinguish the difference between real and performative sex. Hardcore porn becomes sex ed. I've heard far too many accounts of kids as young as six watching porn for the first time. Porn is their first introduction to sex, and because very few young people have access to consent and sex education, their ideas about sex are shaped by porn.

✳ **Porn regularly only shows a specific type of body**: There are some great emerging indie production companies that are showcasing diversity in body shapes, race, gender and ability. However, most mainstream porn exhibits a specific type of body: thin, cis, able-bodied; with large breasts, enormous penises and 'neat' labias. Porn also fetishises, sexualises and objectifies specific minority groups.

✳ **It can normalise sexual aggression**: In sessions with clients, I've tracked a disturbing rise in young women being choked during heterosexual sex without their consent. This is sexual assault. Choking a partner during sex is a popular porn move, and studies suggest that some people are replicating it in real life, thinking it's common practice. This behaviour has been shown to be more common among younger people. And while some people like being choked and consent to it, it is a dangerous and risky sex act if you don't know what you're doing. If all parties involved have not consented and agreed to it, it is sexual assault. It should only ever be done *for* the receiver. If the receiver is not excited by it, then it can be terrifying, traumatising and extremely dangerous.

ETHICAL PORN

Like all things, it's important to consume porn in an ethical way. But the term 'ethical' is much like the term 'all natural ingredients' or 'no nasties' on a packet of lollies. It sounds good, but what does it actually mean? The term 'ethical' is pretty broad, but mostly refers to the ethical production, distribution and consumption of porn. In ethical porn, everyone involved is paid a fair wage, the performers are of legal age, they are consenting and feel safe and respected through the whole process, they consent to you watching the videos, and everyone on set gets a break and can pause at any time. But it could also refer to the type of porn. There might be diversity in bodies, sexuality and sex acts, explicit and ongoing communication, and depictions of safer-sex practices. This doesn't necessarily mean ethical porn has to be romantic – there's heaps of ethical porn that's pretty hardcore too.

The industry is difficult to regulate, so even if content was ethically produced, this would be hard for a user to identify. When I'm speaking with my clients about this, the onus comes back to the consumer to take responsibility for how, where and why they consume ethical porn. Certain companies may liberally slap on the term 'ethical', without practising ethically. If you want to be more ethical in your choices, more often than not you'll need to pay for your porn, in order to ensure that sex workers and performers are paid for the entertainment and art they're creating for you. Research production companies, directors and artists; you can also pay many performers directly via websites or social media.

Sex work is work, so look into how performers or sex workers are getting paid for their service to ensure that the porn you're consuming is ethical. You may also opt for audio porn, or good ol' fashioned erotica.

ARE THERE ANY BENEFITS TO WATCHING PORN?

For adults, there are certainly many good things that can come from ethical, diverse, consensual porn when it is consumed in a mindful, aware and self-regulated way. It can be a great tool to learn how to have sex and to set realistic expectations about bodies. These real depictions of bodies are often censored from mainstream media and porn, so it can actually be an educational and useful exposure to the humanness of sex.

It can be inspiring and sensual as it shows you new ways to touch yourself or your partner, and allows you to witness certain positions, techniques, or experiences that you may not have seen or tried before. It can also be really hot to watch porn with a sexual partner. For this reason, ethical porn can be a fairly safe space to explore fantasies.

Many queer folk say that watching porn was the first time they saw sex scenes that validated their sexuality, like a light bulb moment. They didn't grow up having access to queer love, sex and romance stories, so porn was not only exciting but informative. For them, porn was a cornerstone in their eroticism.

DIFFERENT TYPES OF PORN

Different strokes for different folks. These days there are so many ways to engage with porn, including:

* audio
* erotic stories
* video
* ASMR
* illustration
* images
* art

WHY HAVE MY INTERESTS SHIFTED?

It's not uncommon for your interest in specific genres to shift, change or grow – this happens all the time. For many, their first introduction to porn may have been through videos online, but they've since discovered they prefer the storyline offered in smutty books or audio porn. There are often some fascinating insights into why people seek out different genres, particularly through world events like the pandemic. During lockdowns there was a decrease in searches for content like MILF, stepmum and incest role play porn. Experts suspect this was because people were spending too much time with family, making these fantasies feel a little too close to home. We also saw spikes in searches for public sex, which makes sense – people were fantasising about being able to move freely outdoors again – but the insight that really got my attention was that there was a greater interest in kissing.

As I'm sure you can imagine, 'kissing' isn't usually a key porn search term. This trend was accompanied by a spike in Covid-themed searches for 'medical', 'pandemic' and 'quarantine'. People often seek out porn or fantasies that reflect the spirit or mood of a particular period, or content that allows them to escape the mundane and fantasise about the things they miss and crave. Not only did viewers' interests shift, but the production of the films did too. The Covid safety precautions put in place by independent actors and studios made it functionally impossible to film certain types of sex acts, such as anything that involved a lot of bodily fluids, group sex or anything involving a large group of people in close proximity to each other. In response, more people turned to creating amateur porn at home.

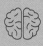 ## Checklist for consuming porn in a more ethical way

* Be clear about your intentions. Is it being used as a stimulus for arousal? Is it for education? Is it to explore fantasies? Is it because you're bored? Is it a habit? Get clear on why you're watching, and ask yourself if it's actually a useful experience.

* Research the site, publication or company to ensure it's run ethically, that the performers and filmmakers are paid fairly, and there are physically and emotionally safe work environments for everyone involved.

* Branch out to different genres. Try audio, novels, illustration or images.

* Pay for your porn.

* Stay present, mindful and aware of your body. Porn can take you out of your body and build arousal more quickly than usual. Try to stay attuned and regulated.

* Examine and challenge whorephobic language used outside of a sexual context; for example, 'you're dressed like a hooker' or 'they're behaving like a porn star'. Degrading sex workers and then consuming their work for free is gross. If you benefit from their work, support their human right to live safely and free from discrimination.

* Notice when, where and how verbal or nonverbal consent is used and reflect on how you feel when it is and isn't present.

* Diversify your viewing habits. Explore beyond the 'top' searches to include diversity in size, race, gender, shape, sexuality, age (adults, being above the age of consent) and ability. You may find something that excites you. Does the site have content for all kinds of viewers beyond the 'male gaze'?

* Opt for scenes where real sex and pleasure are portrayed, in all its messy glory.

IMPORTANT STUFF

✳ People watch porn for pleasure, exploration, stress relief, distraction, inspiration, education and boredom. Whatever it is that drives us to watch porn, undoubtedly the things we watch, read and listen to affect the way we experience sex.

✳ Porn can affect sexual experiences, arousal and pleasure.

✳ Porn isn't created for educational purposes, it is created as entertainment. The intended purpose of porn is to turn you on, stimulate you, arouse your brain and make you climax, and although many people learn about sex through porn, it is rarely created to be educational.

✳ People will never stop watching porn, and we all know that if you tell someone not to do something, it'll only energise the forbidden – but you can consume porn in a more mindful, ethical and self-regulated way.

✳ We're seeing a rise in ethical porn. The term 'ethical' is pretty broad, but mostly refers to the ethical production, distribution and consumption of porn.

✳ When adults consume porn mindfully, ethically and with awareness, it can be a fun way to explore sex, desires and fantasies.

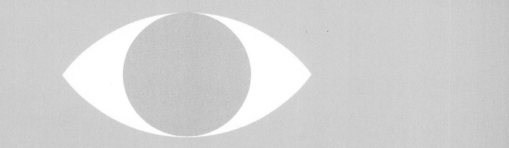

FANTASIES

What do my fantasies say about me? Is it wrong that I think about someone else while I'm having sex? How do I live out my fantasies? Sex theorists and researchers suggest that fantasies exist in the tension between excitement and inhibition. Often, it's the taboo of it all that feels so thrilling. This chapter supports you in exploring your eroticism.

You probably have a sexual fantasy – most of us do. Despite how common they are, talking about fantasies can feel like a revealing and shameful exposure of our innermost desires. It comes down to the perfect combination of wanting something but not knowing if it's okay, plus a sprinkling of the taboo, and the fear that what we desire is perverted or freaky. Fantasising is completely normal and common, but we won't all fantasise about the same thing.

There's an internet meme that says: *Rule 34: if it exists, there's porn made out of it.* The same goes for our fantasies.

Social psychologist Dr Justin Lehmiller identifies seven major themes in fantasies, in his book *Tell Me What You Want*:

* group sex

* power dynamics

* novelty, adventure and variety

* taboo acts

* passion, romance and intimacy

* experimenting with non-monogamy

* experimenting with gender and sexuality.

If your fantasy doesn't fit into those categories, I want to reassure you there's nothing to worry about. They are just seven categories of the more common fantasies. Maybe you're just *really* sexually creative and you can't be put into a little box. I wanted to highlight these categories to prove that you're not the first person to think of something sexual, and you won't be the last. Humans are far more predictable and connected than we think.

There's no right or wrong way to fantasise. If anything, as Dr Lauren Rosewarne, Associate Professor in the School of Social and Political Sciences at the University of Melbourne, says, 'fantasies are a euphemism for daydream'. And if you've ever had a fantasy, which, let's face it, you probably have, you may be curious about what it means, where it comes from, and how to explore and enjoy it safely.

WHY DO I HAVE SEXUAL FANTASIES?

We fantasise for a range of reasons: to build arousal, relieve boredom, escape, relax, feel more sexually confident, and climax. The largest erogenous zone is in between your ears: your brain. The human mind is sexual, creative and exploratory, and fantasising is one very safe way to satisfy our sexual needs and wants. As a result, most people experience a range of enticing, disturbing or challenging sexual fantasies, all of which are normal for most adults, regardless of gender, age or relationship dynamic.

I find that quite often, our fantasies are linked to certain non-sexual desires, past experiences, and even personality traits. For example, a common group sex fantasy has been linked to a desire to feel competent and irresistible.

Of course, that's not to say that's what it means for everyone. Having a sexual fantasy does not always, or even usually, mean that someone is planning to pursue it in real life. It's not necessarily alarming that a lesbian fantasises about having sex with a man, or that someone in a monogamous relationship dreams of their partner being railed by a stranger. Thinking about somebody else while having sex isn't that unusual either and, in most cases, it remains just that – a thought. It may not be cause for concern or damaging to your relationship. Who knows, it might even help to energise the sex you're having. Our imaginations are meant for imagining, after all.

WHAT DO MY SEXUAL FANTASIES MEAN?

Decoding a sexual fantasy is like decoding a dream – difficult and subjective. Our brains often like to categorise and label experiences to make sense of our feelings, rather than just letting us feel what we feel. Sometimes, overthinking a fantasy can remove the allure and taboo. Quite simply, certain things just turn us on. And often there's no rhyme or reason to why you're thinking what you're thinking.

But sometimes it can be useful to examine past experiences and explore core erotic themes, an idea presented by sex therapist Jack Morin in his book *The Erotic Mind.* The concept of core erotic themes engages with the idea that your eroticism is made up of every experience you've ever had, as well as your thoughts, feelings and impulses – the good, the bad and the clunky. In working to explore and understand someone's peak erotic experiences and most arousing fantasies, Morin helps people understand how their past experiences intersect with their fantasies to make sex meaningful.

He also looks at troublesome turn-ons and how people respond when they're at odds with what turns them on. When it comes to troublesome turn-ons, or really anything that's kinky, people are quick to pathologise the taboo. There's often an assumption that the individual has experienced something traumatic and they turn to fantasy as a way to cope, escape, or make something pleasurable that was once painful. For some people, sure, pleasure can be transformational. For example, some recognise that power dynamics have helped them overcome their sexual trauma; they've been able to take back their power. For others, engaging in humiliation play has also helped them heal from being bullied. But this isn't always the case.

A fantasy can be energising because it's a taboo, like when someone says 'don't touch the red button' – of course, we immediately want to touch the red button. It can be arousing to engage in a fantasy that we're not supposed to. However, if it's really troubling you, it may be worth speaking to a professional.

HOW TO EXPLORE YOUR FANTASIES

Exploring your fantasies doesn't necessarily mean *doing them*. It may be as simple as letting your mind wander and exploring what that fantasy might look like, writing about it or masturbating to it. Just because you have a fantasy, doesn't mean you have to live it out (unless you want to! With consent, safety, and pre- and post-sex practices to discuss and unwind after). Keep in mind, not everyone wants to live out or share their fantasies.

A client once asked me, 'How can I make my girlfriend feel comfortable to share her fantasy?' I was really curious about

his use of the word 'make'. He was so set on cultivating a sex-positive and shame-free relationship, where nothing was considered weird or taboo. In theory, this is a useful sentiment, but his girlfriend didn't want to share her fantasies with him – they were for her. He had to recognise that you can't convince, coerce or persuade someone to do, say or share anything they don't want to. And while it may feel like a really intimate or even sexy thing to discuss with your partner, some people just won't feel comfortable revealing this. And that's okay.

Another client fantasised about a mysterious unknown male lover that was completely different from his boyfriend and completely different from his usual type. His most arousing fantasy was about someone else, and even though he didn't want to have sex with anyone else, when he shared this fantasy with his boyfriend it made their sex life complicated. His boyfriend felt disconnected, ashamed, unwanted. They were much happier not knowing where their partner's mind wandered. We worked to rebuild the trust and create boundaries around the type of information that felt useful to share, and the type that didn't.

But I've also seen how some people really get off on sharing their fantasies. One client asked her partner to talk about other women he'd had sex with while she 'fucked' him on top. Another couple would write short erotic novels for each other; every week, they'd share them and then act out the fantasy. And another client said talking about their fantasies was like talking about what they wanted for dinner; sometimes their fantasies aligned and they'd try it, and other times they would unpack them and try to understand why it was such a turn-on.

ARE MY SEXUAL FANTASIES WRONG?

If you're frequently having fantasies about things that are illegal and you want to explore them in real life, I recommend seeking professional support. It can be helpful to have a safe space to discuss and parse out such thoughts. If it's not illegal and all parties are willing and excited about being involved, take a deep breath and get curious. Many people feel ashamed of their turn-ons and inner erotic thoughts, which I'd argue is less constructive, because we bottle them up, which adds tension, and then, well, sometimes they can come out sideways.

Sex is complicated because we can experience both fascination and shame at the same time. Sex can be irrational – things that turn you on don't always make sense. What turns you on might give someone else the ick. And that's normal too. But when we can talk about fantasies, we can understand and value them as an important component of human sexuality. Some fantasies will remain an arousing thought, and others could give you insight into your eroticism and something you want to explore, whether that's with someone else or yourself.

Consider the nature of your most memorable sexual experiences and your most exciting fantasies. Jack Morin describes how the taboo, or something that feels inherently wrong, can energise sex and fantasies through his Erotic Equation: 'Attraction + Obstacle = Excitement'. He believes that although we aspire to a harmonious love life, arousal thrives on the 'dark side of lust'. This is an expression for longing and anticipation, power dynamics, the forbidden and the alluring.

250

YOUR EROTIC MIND

When I was writing this book, I asked people to send in fantasies that I could include. The response was enormous and proved the breadth of human desire and imagination. There were fantasies of being in a Greek temple and seducing an aggressive soldier, hand-feeding a partner with fingers dripping with an ex's cum, fucking multiple people at a swingers' party, being surprised by a partner bringing home another person, getting railed in a grimy nightclub, and being pregnant on a divine queer planet. I don't have enough room to reproduce them all, but here's a taste to whet your palate.

I invite you to read them and notice how your body responds: arousal, intrigue, fear, disgust, excitement, confusion. Look for themes in these desires. Observe where the taboos are present, the existence of the erotic equation and, most importantly, how you feel.

Pansexual, she/her

I'm in the middle of a theatre stage. It's dark everywhere I look, besides a huge light shining on me. I'm surrounded by every ex-boyfriend, lover, sexual partner (all male in this fantasy) I've ever had and they all want to ravish my body sexually. In this fantasy, they're required to physically fight each other. It's chaotic and loud. They beat each other black and blue, they're bleeding, breathing heavily, moaning and yelling. The winner takes me then and there, surrounded by these wounded men. It's the most satisfying, animalistic type of sex. I'd only ever want this as a fantasy, not a reality.

Lesbian, they/she

I want my girlfriend to pick up the hottest woman she can and go home and fuck her like there's no tomorrow. I want her to remember every last detail of the things they do to each other and then tell me while we next fuck. But I also want my girlfriend and me to pick out a guy we both think is cute and take him home and fuck him. Something about two lesbians fucking a man feels very taboo and naughty and makes me so bloody horny.

Straight, he/him

I really enjoy small penis humiliation, although my penis is probably about average. I love the thought of my partner being with another, larger man, getting more pleasure and even insulting me about my inadequacies. The thought of him cumming inside her and stretching her far beyond what I'm capable of really excites me, getting to see her get so much pleasure from it all! Then she would force me to clean it all up, sitting on my face and not letting me move ... And maybe even edging my little cock.

Queer, they/them

I have a housewife fantasy, which feels a bit old-fashioned, but I feel so turned on by the idea of embodying a homemaker role and completely submitting to my man (I think it's more likely a trans guy than a cis guy because I need that emotional intelligence and care!!). The turn-on is providing a beautiful home, meals and space, and not working outside of housework. And then being fucked so good because I've been sooooo good!!!

Pansexual, he/him

My fantasy is to take part in a threesome FFM or MMF. I'd love for the other male participant to be a workmate of mine who's very fit, and I can imagine him being well-endowed like myself. I would love to have sex with my wife and him in our home. My fantasy is to have anal sex with my wife while at the same time sucking off my workmate. If the third person was female I would love her to have a strap-on and satisfy my wife while I am behind her, working her butt. The peak moment would be having the third person behind me; they'd jerk me off on my wife's face and drip my warm cum on my wife's tongue and cheeks. Then I'd clean up her mouth and face with my mouth.

Straight, she/her

I often fantasise about alien or creature forced impregnation. It's the taboo of a creature taking control and using a female human as a breeding vessel. This is just in porn – I don't fantasise about this during sex or ask sexual partners to enact it. I'm also aware that non-consensual sex is wrong in real life, and I don't even want children. The fantasy just turns me on!

Straight, she/her

I'm at a sexy older man's place, I'm sitting on the edge of a table. His hands trail down to my vagina, which is already sopping wet, and he runs his fingers over it before gently coaxing himself inside and finding my perfect spot. He whispers, 'I can tell you haven't had your body praised before.' He keeps working me with his fingers until I tell him to stop because I'm about to cum, but I want to do it on his dick. He teases me with the tip of his dick around the entrance to my vagina until he starts sliding in, painstakingly slow, so I can feel absolutely every inch he gains as I hold on to him. I tell him that I'm going to cum and he begs for it, saying that he can take it, and I know he means that I can throw all of myself at him and be safe, so I cum and then cum even harder as he does at the same time.

Bisexual, she/her

I have this fantasy of being the other woman, specifically with someone who's married, someone who's so into me that they can't help themselves. I feel like the sex would be so hot because it's forbidden. But I think the reason I find this so hot is because I don't actually have to commit to this person, and I can just fantasise about it without actually hurting someone.

Bisexual, she/they

My fantasies are often gender-bendy, where people's bodies and genitals change. My boyfriend is fucking me and then my vulva transforms into a penis and I watch my boyfriend suck on it and I fuck him in the arse. It's hot because it's an array of experiences in the one session. I also fantasise that I'm in the body of someone with a penis fucking myself and imagining how it would feel to fuck me. I like imagining how good and sexy my body might feel to someone else.

Straight, she/her

I have a fantasy of pegging a guy. My interest was sparked through watching prostate-milking pornographic videos, and the fascination has stuck – to the extent that I even purchased myself an entry-level strap-on a couple of years ago. I live in a regional town where monogamous, heteronormative relationships are the most accepted form of relationship, boys are brought up to have very 'masculine' interests and any mention of anal play among men is seen as 'gay'. This homophobic rhetoric is what leads me to the 'taboo' of anal play with the men I meet. I want to really fuck them. But I have no actual desire to fulfil it.

Bi-curious he/him

My deepest fantasy is to be in a bi threesome. Just the thought of being fucked by a big cock while I eat a pussy and then DP with the woman gets me so hot and bothered. I'm getting hard typing this, and it's all just a big old fantasy as I'm in a relationship with a woman I love but who isn't a kinky mofo like me.

Bisexual she/her

A male vampire and male fae fuck a powerful female fae. I never thought I would be into MMF threesomes, but, oh my god, the vampire behind her stimulating her clit and biting at her neck and holding her up while the other fae male is fucking her – and they're in a cave and it's so sexy and tender and passionate and the moonlight is shining in on them. As a woman, the idea of being worshipped by two men is incredibly arousing and I imagine some fuck buddies doing that for real and I am surprised at how turned on I am, how curious I am to try.

Straight he/him

I am turned on by women when they sweat. Their hair gets all curly and nasty, their skin starts glowing and the sweat pools up at the best places (neck, collarbone, cleavage and lower back). The salty smell of sweat mixed with their perfume is almost intoxicating to me. One time, when a partner of mine came back from her workout, the way she looked just made me go feral. I tried experiencing this solo by listening to naughty audios involving a gym trainer who makes a move on her client after a workout. It was awesome. I tried out this fantasy with a partner and it was probably the best foreplay and sex I've ever had.

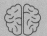

Write your fantasy down

Now it's your go. In as much detail as possible, describe your most arousing fantasy. Think about the context, location, the time of year, details about where you are and who you are. Describe who it's for, any supporting characters, emotions or feelings present, sexual acts, elements of taboo, the peak moment of pleasure. Be descriptive and explicit.

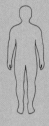

Feel into your fantasy

Read over your fantasy, now place it somewhere away from you. Take a few minutes to feel into your body. What are you noticing? Is there a physical, emotional, mental or erotic response? After a few moments, feel into whether the activity is complete or whether you'd like to continue exploring your fantasy through writing, masturbating or sex with other people.

IMPORTANT STUFF

✳ Eroticism and our fantasies make sex meaningful. It isn't necessarily the act of sex. Rather, it is a process of imagination and expression that is a result of your unique human experience. .

✳ Our erotic landscape includes but isn't limited to thoughts, impulses and desires, and is connected to all aspects of life, some pleasurable and others not.

✳ Some people will want to experience their fantasies, but others are happy for them to live in their imagination.

✳ A fantasy can be energising because it's a taboo; it can be arousing to engage in a fantasy that we're not supposed to. The taboo energises our sexual experiences.

✳ Sex is complicated because we can experience both fascination and shame at the same time. Sex can be irrational – things that turn you on don't always make sense.

✳ Understanding your fantasies can be intriguing, useful, arousing and at times disturbing. But taking the time to reflect, explore and feel into your fantasies may lead to a greater awareness of your sexuality and more-fulfilling sex.

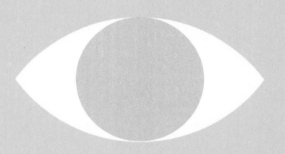

A final word

The intention of this book is to bring together some of the foundational tools I offer in session. As I was writing, it just kept getting bigger. Much like how I feel about pleasure, I wanted more. To the dismay of my editor and my clenched jaw, I wrote more than double the words we'd agreed on. I said in the introduction that sex was fucking huge and, yeah, I really proved that to myself. Despite it blowing out, there's also so much I didn't get to. And despite this process feeling like childbirth (*this is purely anecdotal because I actually haven't done this yet), I'm already forgetting the pain and I want to go back for seconds. So maybe there will be another book one day.

There aren't too many books written by those who have training in the somatics, largely because many of them are more interested in spending time in their bodies, and, fuck me, sitting at a desk writing for a year isn't what I'd originally thought of as a true embodied experience. But through this book, my mind and body processed a lot – heartbreak, death, grief, starting a new life, falling in love. Everything that went into this book was more somatic than I ever thought it could be.

I started working on this book a week after I separated from my partner of six years. Heartbreak is a painful, full-body experience, one I know many of us have felt. I developed a habit of waking up at 3 am and felt such severe pain I didn't know how to move or think. I fell into my network of supportive friends and family, who always answered my calls, and took up 6 am ocean plunges in winter to shock my nervous system. I moved my body every day to self-regulate, and got really comfortable with crying in public, receiving many generous looks from strangers that I took to mean, 'Don't worry, it always gets better.'

I did hours of therapy, and mostly I threw myself into work. I'm by no means recommending this approach – it led to late-stage burnout at the end of the year – but working, researching, reading and writing about sex gave me purpose and drive. This would be a very different book if I'd written it the year before my break-up, and no doubt it'd be different if I wrote it years from now too. I had to put into practice all the tools and approaches I'd shared with my own clients over the years and had some of the most profound, memorable, full-body experiences of pleasure. I was humbly reminded of the intense vulnerability that new experiences require, which filled me with empathy and awe for my clients, who consistently show up in session after reaching their own learning edges. I learnt by doing, because I practised everything I've put in this book, over and over again.

The way we understand sex, relationships and bodies is changing at a rapid pace. There is more information, research and resources about sex than ever before. And in this process of change we will continue to grow. The way we understand sex as a collective and as individuals will be very different in a few years. We're always changing. With all of the words and all of the practices written in this book, there's only one thing to remember: you learn by doing.

You will learn about what you want, and how to ask for it, by doing.

You will overcome fear, shame and anxiety, by doing.

You will experience more pleasure, by doing.

We can't just read or think our way to good sex, we need to experience it, on our own or with others. And it is in the experience that you will change. Now here I am, handing it all over to you. Take what you want and leave the rest. Pleasure is your responsibility, so go get it.

Sources

Chapter 1

'being queer' not as being about who you're having sex with: bell hooks, 'Bell Hooks – Are You Still a Slave? Liberating the Black Female Body I Eugene Lang College', The New School, YouTube video, 6 May 2014.

Chapter 2

Window of tolerance: Daniel Siegel, *The Developing Mind*, Guildford Press, 1999.

Chapter 3

Pleasure is a measure of freedom: Adrienne Maree Brown on *The Laura Flanders Show*, YouTube video, 14 May 2019.
Body positivity started as a social movement: Helana Darwin & Amara Miller, 'Factions, frames, and postfeminism(s) in the Body Positive Movement', *Feminist Media Studies*, 2021, vol.21, no.6, pp.873–90.
Failing to acknowledge body positivity's radical past: Amanda Mull, 'Body positivity is a scam', *Vox*, 5 Jun 2018.
Great lovers aren't born, they're made: Peggy Kleinplatz in Don Butler, 'Extraordinary sex for boomers: Great lovers are made, not born, expert says', *Ottawa Citizen*, 8 Oct 2014.
The feelings wheel: Dr Gloria Willcox, 'The feelings wheel: unlock the power of your emotions', Calm, www.calm.com/blog/the-feelings-wheel
Participants drew maps of body locations: Lauri Nummenmaa et al., 'Bodily maps of emotions', *Psychological and Cognitive Sciences*, 2013, vol.111, no.2, pp.646–51.
The stronger the feeling is physically: Lauri Nummenmaa et al., 'Maps of subjective feelings', *Biological Sciences*, 2018, vol.115, no.37, pp.9198–9203.

Chapter 4

The first in-depth study of the clitoris: Helen E O'Conell et al., 'Anatomical relationship between urethra and clitoris', *Journal of Urology*, vol.159, Jun 1998, pp.1892–1897.
Sheri Winston coined the 'groove tube': Sheri Winston, *Women's Anatomy of Arousal*, Mango Garden Press, 2010.
A 'handbrake': Emily Nagoski, *Come as You Are*, Simon & Schuster, 2015, p.49.
Arousal non-concordance is the well-established phenomenon: ibid.

Chapter 6

Masters and Johnson's Phases of the Sexual Response Cycle: William Masters & Virginia Johnson, *Human Sexual Response*, Bantam Books, 1966.
Kaplan's Triphasic Model of Sexual Response: Helen Kaplan, *Disorders of Sexual Desire and Other New Concepts and Techniques in Sex Therapy*, Brunner/Hazel Publications, 1979.
Awakening sensation in the hands: Betty Martin, 'Waking up your hands', bettymartin.org/hands
Between 20 to 30 per cent of men experience PE: Christopher Martin et al., 'Current and emerging therapies in premature ejaculation: where we are coming from, where we are going', *International Journal of Urology*, vol.24, Issue 1, Jan 2017, pp.40–50.
A study found that 82 per cent of men who suffered lifelong premature ejaculation: Antonio L Pastore et al., 'Pelvic floor muscle rehabilitation for patients with lifelong premature ejaculation: a novel therapeutic approach', *Therapeutic Advances in Urology*, 2014, vol.6, no.3, pp.83–88.

Chapter 7

Have sex in a way that leaves everyone involved: Jaclyn Friedman, 'Sex & Consent: it's time to go beyond the rules', Refinery 29, online article, 6 Sep 2018.
As a legal reform, this is monumental: Chanel Contos, *Consent Laid Bare*, Pan Macmillan, 2023, p.72.

Chapter 9
Pee after sex to minimise the chances of a urinary tract infection: Planned Parenthood, 'Urinary tract infections (UTIs)', www.plannedparenthood.org/learn/health-and-wellness/urinary-tract-infections-utis
One in six people will get an STI: BetterHealth channel, 'Everybody's doing it!', www.betterhealth.vic.gov.au/campaigns/sti-testing-week
Open conversations around sexual health actively lessen the risk of STI transmission: Hildie Leung et al., 'Development of contextually-relevant sexuality education: Lessons from a comprehensive review of adolescent sexuality education across cultures', *International Journal of Environmental Research and Public Health*, 2019, vol.16, no.4, p.621.
People who disclose their STI to their partners have more positive feelings: Julia E. Hood & Allison L. Friedman, 'Unveiling the hidden epidemic: A review of stigma associated with sexually transmissible infections', *Sex Health*, June 2011, vol.8, no.2, pp.159–70.

Chapter 10
Foreplay starts at the end of the previous orgasm: Esther Perel, X, 14 Jan 2016.

Chapter 11
A drive is a biological mechanism: Emily Nagoski, op. cit. p.229.

Chapter 12
Skene's glands are the source of ejaculation in people with vulvas: Cleveland Clinic, 'Skene's gland', my.clevelandclinic.org/health/body/24089-skenes-gland
Inhaled nitrite is a liquid drug that gives a high, spaced out, dizzy feeling: Frank Romanelli et al., 'Poppers: epidemiology and clinical management of inhaled nitrite abuse', *Pharmacotherapy*, Jan 2004, issue 24, no.1, pp.69–78.

3 per cent having learnt about safe LGBTQIA+ sex in school: Big Australian Sex Survey 2022, NORMAL, itsnormal.com/pages/big-sex-survey-2022

Chapter 14
The positive impact vibrator use can have on sexual arousal and function: Debra Herbenick et al., 'Prevalence and characteristics of vibrator use by women in the United States: Results from a nationally representative study', *Journal of Sexual Medicine*, 6, 2009, pp.1857–1866.
A majority of people don't experience any genital symptoms: Debra Herbenick et al., ibid.

Chapter 16
Self-perceived porn addiction ... is not a formally recognised disorder: Athena Duffy et al., 'Pornography addiction in adults: A systematic review of definitions and reported impact', *Journal of Sexual Medicine*, May 2016, vol.13, no.5.
It was difficult to pinpoint at what point pornography use became addiction: Rubén de Alarcón et al., 'Online porn addiction: what we know and what we don't—a systematic review', *Journal of Clinical Medicine*, 2019; vol.8, no.1.

Chapter 17
Dr Justin Lehmiller identifies seven major themes in fantasies: Justin Lehmiller, 'The 7 most common sex fantasies – and how many people have ever had them', *Sex and Psychology*, blog post, 13 Mar 2019.
Fantasies are a euphemism for daydream: Dr Lauren Rosewarne in 'Why you should make your sexual fantasy a reality', *In Bed* podcast, Feb 2022.
Attraction + Obstacle = Excitement: Jack Morin, *The Erotic Mind*, HarperCollins, 1995, p.50.

Acknowledgements

This book is not a solo act. Its creation has been a collective process that spans across generations of thinking and feeling.

I want to start by acknowledging the many pleasure activists, educators, researchers, sex workers, LGBTQIA+ advocates, therapists, writers and artists, who have created a world where we can speak more freely about pleasure, who've informed the way we teach now, who have fought for change and justice even in the threat of their own safety, who have created community and spaces where we can gather to learn, who have inspired not only the way I work and teach but the way I move through the world.

To my clients and those who have trusted me over the years, in sessions and workshops. Thank you for your vulnerability, and thank you for allowing me to be at those learning edges with you. You have inspired this book.

Deej Juventin, everything useful I've learnt about therapy, sex, relationships and trauma is from you. Thank you for your congruence and knowledge, and your capacity to keep me, and many, at a learning edge. You have ruptured and repaired the way I understand systems of learning; I am so grateful to have had access to you. And thank you for your big, camp laugh.

A very special thanks to Mark Campbell. I really didn't think I could write a book until I met you. Or at least I was too scared to. You've held my hand with an entwined finger grip through this whole process. Thank you for your intuition and feeling; your somatic knowledge has guided this book to where it needs to be. Madeleine James, Vanessa Lanaway, Susan McCreery and the whole HarperCollins team, you are so consistent and thorough and brilliant. Thank you for being able to step back and make it make sense.

Meredith Jansen, your illustrations gave this book a pulse. Thank you for working with me to bring the colour, joy, wet-hot pleasure and diversity that sex ed deserves. Mietta Yans, it's like you crawled into my brain and skin and knew exactly how to design this book, and thank god you did because I could never have done this without you. Your design is essential to the learning and feeling experience of it all. Working with artists and a creative team has been vital to normalise pleasure and remove shame and fear from sex ed.

Ben Grand, you dream really big and you make it happen.

To a notable team of people I have learnt from and with, Deej Juvenintin (you again), Uma Ayelet, Tanya Koens, Dr Betty Martin, Dr Martha Lee and my supervision group, Aleks Trkjulia, Arlyn Owen, Christine Rafe, Jack Martin and Kass Mourikis. Your expertise and skill has challenged and inspired me, and has been foundational for the moments I've felt most stuck. Lucy Wark, you're the business and the pleasure, thank you for your research and your hyperfixation on making sex ed accessible. Sarah Frish, for your skill, wit and your taste, and years of turning big lofty ideas into tangible resources.

I want to acknowledge and thank Dr Betty Martin for reviewing and approving the use of the Three-minute Game and The Wheel of Consent in this book.

Demon Derriere, thank you for the way you inspired, challenged and transformed ideas in this book. You are a force that is so strong and warm. Thank you for the way you create community and spaces of joy. You, my friend, are a gift.

Rashida Dungarwalla, the congruence, care and insight you offered when we worked together to create body confidence resources has had an enduring impact on the way I support clients and the tools I have shared in this book. Thank you.

Audre Lorde, Adrienne Maree Brown, bell hooks, Betty Dodson, Jack Morin, Emily Nagoski: I'd choose to have dinner with you.

To all my friends who are the loves of my life, I feel like I'm doing pretty well because I've got you. You've been a kickstand when I've felt wobbly. Platonic love is what I live for.

Mum, Dad, Al, Dan and Em and my whole family. Growing up with a foundation of safety and love has made doing challenging things feel okay. I've always had you.

To Harriet, thank you for your love and your wisdom and your ideas and grounded vision, you were my reminder to stay in the process. I found you when I was writing this book, and I also found me.

And of course, to you. To your mind and your body. Thank you for your openness and reflection. Thank you for reading something edgy, for the time you've spent practising, feeling uncomfortable and doing things differently. I hope your enquiry goes well beyond this book and I hope you've found pleasure.

263

The sex menu: what's your pleasure?

If you're like every human ever, sometimes it's easier to suss out what you actually want or are curious about when you can feel into the options. This is where a sex menu can be really useful. It can help you explore new things, gauge curiosity from yourself and others and create space for communication. The sex menu I've created for you on the following pages may help you externalise your desires and remove the pressure to come up with all the possibilities by yourself, equipping you to talk about anything that feels useful with future sexual partners.

Type of sexual experience	Yes	No	I need more information
69			
Abstinence			
Aftercare			
Amateur porn			
Anal massage			
Anal penetration			
Anal play			
Audio porn			
Blindfolds			
Breathwork			
Butt plugs			
Casual sex			
Clit stimulation			
Condoms			
Couples therapy			
Dating			

Type of sexual experience	Yes	No	I need more information
Dental dam			
Dirty talk			
Dominance			
Dry humping			
Edging			
Electrostimulation			
Erogenous zones			
Erotic writing			
Feet play			
Fingering			
Fisting			
Flirting			
Food play			
Foreplay			
Friends with benefits			
Fucking			
Gagging			
Genital gazing			
Golden shower			
Group sex			
Hand job			
Hand play			
Hugs			
Impact play			
Intimacy			
Kegels			
Kink/BDSM			

Type of sexual experience	Yes	No	I need more information
Kissing			
Loud sex			
Lube			
Mapping: body/genitals			
Massage			
Masturbation			
Me on top			
Mindful sex			
Mirror work			
Mutual masturbation			
Nipple/chest/breast play			
Nipple play			
One-night stand			
Open relationship			
Oral			
Other on top			
Outercourse			
Penetrative sex			
Penis play			
Period sex			
Phone sex			
Power play			
Punishing			
Rimming			
Role play			
Safe words			
Scissoring			
Sending nudes			

Type of sexual experience	Yes	No	I need more information
Sensate focus			
Sensation play			
Sensual eating			
Sensual massage			
Sex in public			
Sex party			
Sex work			
Sexting			
Shower/bath			
Slow sex			
Spanking			
Spooning			
Squirting			
Strap-on			
Strip tease			
Submission			
Swinging			
Tantra			
Teasing			
Threesome			
Tickling			
Toys			
Voyeurism			
Vulva play			
Watching porn			
Wax play			
Whip			
Witnessing/being witnessed			

Glossary

AFAB Assigned female at birth.

Ally A person who supports and advocates for the rights and wellbeing of LGBTQIA+ individuals.

AMAB Assigned male at birth.

Androgynous Having a combination of masculine and feminine traits in appearance or behaviour.

Aromantic An individual who does not experience romantic attraction towards others.

Asexual A sexual orientation characterised by a lack of sexual attraction or desire towards others.

ASMR Autonomous sensory meridian response is a physical and psychological response to auditory, visual or tactile stimulus. ASMR can be used to relax, feel good, reduce stress and even arouse.

BDSM An acronym referring to bondage, discipline/dominance, submission/sadism or masochism.

Benching When someone keeps a potential romantic interest on hold, stringing them along without fully committing.

Bigender Individuals who identify as having two genders simultaneously or alternating between two genders.

Bisexual An individual who is attracted to more than one gender.

Breadcrumbing When someone gives intermittent or minimal attention or communication to a romantic interest to maintain their interest without fully committing.

Brotherboy A term used by First Nations people to describe gender-diverse people who have a male spirit and take on male roles within the community.

Catfishing The act of creating a false online identity to deceive someone, often for romantic or emotional purposes.

Cisgender Commonly referred to as cis, describes individuals whose gender identity aligns with the sex assigned to them at birth.

Coming out The process of sharing one's sexual orientation or gender identity to others. For many it is a pivotal point in their sexual and gender identity, for others it is not. Not all people feel comfortable, safe or even want to 'come out'.

Commitment phobia The fear or avoidance of long-term commitment or serious relationships.

Compersion Loosely refers to experiencing happiness when your partner is connecting romantically or sexually with another person. A great analogy for this is when your partner gets a promotion, or your best friend goes on a great date. Even though it's not your experience, you're happy for them.

Consent Verbal and nonverbal communication that ascertains everyone is excited, willing and/or wanting to engage in a specific sexual activity

Cuffing season The time during colder months when people seek out a partner for the purpose of cosying up and keeping warm.

Demisexual Someone who experiences sexual attraction only after forming a strong emotional connection with another person.

Drag The performance art of dressing in clothing typically associated with an expression of a different gender from the artist's.

Dry humping Where you grind against your partner, with clothes on, to increase sensation and arousal.

DTF Down to Fuck

Emotional availability The ability to be open, receptive and present in emotional interactions and relationships.

Emotional intelligence The ability to understand, manage and express emotions effectively, both within oneself and in relationships with others.

Fantasy Imagined or desired sexual scenarios or experiences that may or may not be acted upon.

Foreplay Moments to connect, build arousal and sync up your nervous systems before sex.

FWB Friends With Benefits, referring to a relationship where individuals engage in casual sexual activity without a romantic commitment.

Gender dysphoria Discomfort or distress experienced by an individual when their gender identity does not align with the sex they were assigned at birth.

Genderqueer An umbrella term for individuals who do not identify exclusively as male or female.

Ghosting When someone suddenly cuts off all communication with a romantic partner or potential interest without explanation.

Greysexual/grey ace An individual who experiences limited sexual attraction, or only under certain circumstances.

Heteronormative Denoting or relating to a world view that promotes heterosexuality as the normal or preferred sexual orientation; the assumption that heterosexuality is the norm or default sexual orientation.

Heterosexual An individual who is attracted to people of a different gender.

Homosexual An individual who is attracted to people of the same gender.

Intercourse Sexual activity involving penetration, typically referring to vaginal or anal sex.

Intersex A general term used for a variety of situations in which a person is born with reproductive or sexual anatomy that doesn't fit in the boxes of 'female' or 'male'.

Jealousy A complex emotion characterised by feelings of insecurity, fear or resentment in response to a perceived threat to a romantic relationship.

Kink Anything beyond the straight and narrow; various sexual practices or desires that are considered unconventional, often involving power dynamics, role playing or fetishes.

LGBTQIA+ An acronym representing a diverse range of sexual orientations and gender identities: lesbian, gay, bisexual, transgender, queer, intersex, asexual, and the plus is inclusive of other identities.

Love bombing A manipulative tactic where someone overwhelms another person with excessive attention, affection and grand gestures in order to gain control or manipulate their emotions.

Love language The way in which a person expresses and receives love, such as through acts of service, words of affirmation, quality time, physical touch or receiving gifts.

Love triangle A situation where three people are romantically involved or interested in each other, often leading to complex emotional dynamics.

Lubricant A substance used to reduce friction and enhance comfort during sexual activities, such as water-based or silicone-based lubricants.

Masturbation Sexual self-stimulation, usually to attain sexual pleasure or release.

Monogamy The practice of having a single romantic or sexual partner at a time.

Non-binary Individuals who do not identify exclusively as male or female.

Open relationship A relationship where one or both partners agree to have sexual or romantic connections with other people.

Orgasm The peak of sexual pleasure, often accompanied by muscle contractions and pleasurable sensations.

Outercourse Any sexual activity or experience that happens outside the body, i.e. toys, kissing, touch, massage. The term 'outercourse' is used instead of 'foreplay', as the term 'foreplay' suggests acts like oral are done before the main event of penetration. Outercourse is just as pleasurable and valid as intercourse.

Pansexual An individual who is attracted to people regardless of their gender identity or biological sex.

PDA An acronym for 'public display of affection', referring to physical displays of affection between partners in public.

Polyamory The practice of having multiple, consensual and ethical romantic or sexual relationships.

Polysexual An individual who is attracted to multiple genders, but not necessarily all genders.

Queer An umbrella term used to encompass diverse sexual orientations and gender identities outside of societal norms.

Questioning Individuals who are exploring and questioning their sexual orientation or gender identity.

Relationship anarchy A philosophy that rejects hierarchical and predefined relationship structures, emphasising autonomy, consent and individual needs.

Relationship goals A term used to describe the aspirational qualities or achievements that people desire in their romantic relationships.

Relationship milestones Significant events or achievements that mark progress or growth in a romantic relationship, such as moving in together, getting a love fern, introducing them to your friends and family.

Safer sex Engaging in sexual activities while taking precautions to prevent unwanted pregnancies and sexually transmitted infections (STIs).

Sapiosexual Someone who is attracted to intelligence or intellectual qualities in others.

Sexual arousal The physiological changes that happen in your body as a result of something stimulating you.

Sexual orientation One's enduring pattern of emotional, romantic and/or sexual attraction.

Sex positions Various ways individuals can engage in sexual activities, like missionary, doggy style or 69.

Sexual wellness Taking care of one's sexual health through regular check-ups, practising safer sex and maintaining healthy relationships.

Sexuality Refers to an individual's sexual orientation, attractions, desires and behaviours.

Sexually transmitted infections (STIs) Infections spread through sexual contact, such as chlamydia, gonorrhoea, herpes or HIV/AIDS.

Sistergirl A term used by First Nations people to describe gender-diverse people that have a female spirit and take on female roles within the community.

Slow fade When someone gradually reduces communication and interaction with a romantic partner or potential interest, often without explicitly ending the relationship.

Soulmates The belief that there is a special person or people with whom one is destined to have a deep and meaningful connection.

Transgender Individuals whose gender identity does not align with the sex assigned to them at birth.

U-haul lesbian A stereotype of women in same-sex or lesbian relationships who move in together after a short period of time. It suggests an inclination to committed relationships.

Vibrator A device used for sexual pleasure that produces vibrations to stimulate erogenous zones.

Whorephobia A term used to describe prejudice, discrimination or negative attitudes towards individuals who engage in sex work or the sex-work industry. It refers to any beliefs or actions that stigmatise, devalue or marginalise sex workers based on their profession.

Harper *by* Design

An imprint of HarperCollins*Publishers*

HarperCollins*Publishers*
Australia · Brazil · Canada · France · Germany · Holland · India
Italy · Japan · Mexico · New Zealand · Poland · Spain · Sweden
Switzerland · United Kingdom · United States of America

HarperCollins acknowledges the Traditional Custodians
of the lands upon which we live and work, and pays respect
to Elders past and present.

First published on Gadigal Country in Australia in 2024
by HarperCollins*Publishers* Australia Pty Limited
ABN 36 009 913 517
harpercollins.com.au

A catalogue record for this book is available from the National Library of Australia

ISBN 978 1 4607 6537 1 (hardback)
ISBN 978 1 4607 1716 5 (ebook)

Publisher: Mark Campbell
Publishing Director: Brigitta Doyle
Project editor: Madeleine James
Cover and internal design by Mietta Yans, HarperCollins Design Studio
Illustrations by Meredith Jensen
Colour reproduction by Splitting Image Colour Studio, Wantirna, Victoria
Printed and bound in China by 1010 Printing

8 7 6 5 4 3 2 1   24 25 26 27 28

About the author

Georgia Grace is a certified sex and relationship practitioner and somatic therapist who is particularly known for her work in somatic sexology, embodied counselling and trauma-informed practices. Her approach to working with sex and relationships is inclusive, sex-positive and shame-free, and supports individuals, couples and groups to overcome common sexual concerns. She is also a co-founder of NORMAL, a sexual wellness company, where she works with Lucy Wark and a team of experts to create educational courses and design modern sex toys. Georgia is a regular contributor to a variety of top-tier media outlets as a writer, speaker and podcaster. She is on a mission to redefine what 'normal' means when it comes to sex, relationships and intimacy, and equip people with the tools they need to address these typically taboo topics for more fulfilling experiences.

georgiagrace.co

@gspot._